Muslim and Catholic Responses to HIV and AIDS in Kenya

Ethnographies of Religion

Series Editor
Peter Marina, University of Wisconsin–La Crosse

As religion pushes toward an uncertain late-modern world rife with contradictions, and as modern rationality unevenly blends with supernatural beliefs, this series will focus on spatial and temporal practices of embodied religious experience in the (post)modern world. Works in the series will move beyond the hard world of maps and demographics of researchers who chart the quantitative spread of religions, and into religious spaces and places where people actively make meanings and responses to their structural conditions. Taking seriously the assertion of Michele de Certeau that "what maps cut up, the story cuts across," this book series looks for creative ethnographic styles to travel the soft, malleable, and bending spaces with those engaged in religious practices as it occurs in time and space. The importance of connecting history, structure, culture, and biography offers insight into the dialectical role of religion in the modern world, one that is expected to yield highly surprising results. The ethnographic approaches taken throughout this series will take into account the public and private spaces of religious experience where the visible and invisible, mundane and transcendent, ecstatic and frightful, and myopic and reflexive worlds burst from the scenes of social life into the pages of this series.

Recent Titles in Series

Muslim and Catholic Responses to HIV and AIDS in Kenya, by Timothy James Carey

Religious Vitality in Christian Intentional Communities: A Comparative Ethnographic Study, by Mark Killian

Muslim and Catholic Responses to HIV and AIDS in Kenya

Timothy James Carey

LEXINGTON BOOKS
Lanham • Boulder • New York • London

Published by Lexington Books
An imprint of The Rowman & Littlefield Publishing Group, Inc.
4501 Forbes Boulevard, Suite 200, Lanham, Maryland 20706
www.rowman.com

Unit A, Whitacre Mews, 26-34 Stannary Street, London SE11 4AB

British Library Cataloguing in Publication Information Available

Library of Congress Cataloging-in-Publication Data

Names: Carey, Timothy James, author.
Title: Muslim and Catholic responses to HIV and AIDS in Kenya / Timothy James Carey.
Description: Lanham : Lexington Books, 2018. | Series: Ethnographies of religion | Includes bibliographical references and index.
Identifiers: LCCN 2018028678 (print) | LCCN 2018030523 (ebook) | ISBN 9781498578295 (Electronic) | ISBN 9781498578288 (cloth : alk. paper)
Subjects: LCSH: AIDS (Disease)--Patients--Care--Kenya. | Care of the sick--Religious aspects--Christianity. | Care of the sick--Religious aspects--Islam. | AIDS (Disease)--Religious aspects--Christianity. | AIDS (Disease)--Religious aspects--Islam.
Classification: LCC RA643.86.K4 (ebook) | LCC RA643.86.K4 C373 2018 (print) | DDC 362.1969792096762--dc23
LC record available at https://lccn.loc.gov/2018028678

∞™ The paper used in this publication meets the minimum requirements of American National Standard for Information Sciences Permanence of Paper for Printed Library Materials, ANSI/NISO Z39.48-1992.

Printed in the United States of America

Contents

Preface

The present research seeks to situate the contemporary discourse regarding HIV and AIDS in Nairobi, Kenya, in a specific sociohistorical and religious moment. Many competing and conflicting elements create the complex web of identity there, chief among them, confessional religious, political, and ethnic identity markers, to name but a few. As a researcher, I chose to offer this snapshot of popular views regarding HIV and AHDS among the Catholic and Sunni Muslim population of Kenya's capital city by interviewing religious leadership with the implicit assumption that these leaders have a significant impact on public opinion within their respective communities of faith and can even help to shape general views of the virus.

Employing social scientific research methods, I strove to maintain impartiality on the topic, opting to let the leaders present their own views on certain issues related to the epidemic. Yet, as a theologian who himself is largely concerned with issues of social justice, I now realize that the document itself exhibits an internal theology that favors justice over stigma, dignity over exclusion from the common good, and a conceptual openness toward the religious other in pursuit of an interreligious dialogue that can affirm the inherent humanity of those negatively affected by HIV and AIDS.

In this way, I am biased since I perceive the beneficial and dynamic dimensions of both religious traditions to create and positively transform society into one that nurtures all members of its community and affords a privileged place for the poor, the sick, and the needy, and which is informed by a commitment to justice, mercy, and hospitality. I hope that the reader will agree.

Abbreviations

ABC	Abstain, be faithful, use a condom
AIC	African independent churches
AIDS	Acquired immunodeficiency syndrome
ART	Antiretroviral therapy
AZT	Azidothymidine
FBO	Faith-based organization
CIA	Central Intelligence Agency (USA)
CBO	Community-based organization
CCAWT	Circle of Concerned African Women Theologians
CDC	Centers for Disease Control and Prevention (USA)
FGM	Female genital mutilation
HIV	Human immunodeficiency virus
IDU	Intravenous drug use
IRE	Islamic religious education
KAIS	Kenyan AIDS Indicator Survey
KCI	Kenyan Council of Imams
KD	Kairos Document
KEC	Kenyan Episcopal Conference
MTCT	Mother-to-child transmission
NACC	National AIDS Control Council (Kenya)

NGO	Non-governmental organization
PEPFAR	President's Emergency Plan for AIDS Relief (USA)
PLHIV	People living with HIV
PLWHA	People living with HIV or AIDS
SUPKEM	Supreme Council of Kenyan Muslims
UNAIDS	Joint United National Programme on HIV/AIDS
VCT	Voluntary counseling and testing
WHO	World Health Organization

Introduction

"Remove the harm, Lord of Men, and give healing": Muslim and Catholic Responses to HIV and AIDS in Kenya

INTRODUCTION AND PLAN FOR THE CHAPTER

"As Thomas Aquinas and Josef Fuchs often remind us," write James F. Keenan, SJ and Jon Fuller, SJ, "the descent into the particular is always an encounter with more and more variables."[1] Religion means a great many things to a great many people. As a matter of good methodology, theologians must indicate explicitly and exactly what we mean when we speak or write on a given topic. Otherwise, we run the risk of getting bogged down in unknown territories that yield little fruit, or we get stuck in minutiae that becomes an enormous project of its own. Or, worse yet, we end up trying to write about a topic on which we are unqualified. Navigating these pitfalls—amongst others—can be a daunting task, yet it has its own distinct satisfaction and reward.

It is the responsibility of the theologian to faithfully treat the material under consideration. This project begins with the methodological presupposition that the religious traditions of Sunni Islam and African Catholicism are useful topics for comparison since they bridge the human and the divine worlds. That is, these religious traditions, rooted firmly in their own theologies, forms of scripture, and doctrine—are also formed by the human societies within which they practically exist expressed in ritual and practice.[2] Further, these religious traditions produce certain observable patterns of organization and behavior as a basic human necessity. As a comparativist, I find these patterns to be attractive foci for analysis to see why humans act in the way they do. However, far from arguing that this data is objectively quantifiable, I instead posit that these patterns constitute an insightful, descriptive account into how persons religious understand themselves and the world they inhabit.[3]

The chapter proceeds in this way. Each of the succeeding sections explores a major issue or question dealing with the practical methodology adopted for this project. Beginning with an explanation of the fieldwork undertaken for this research, the chapter then considers why the two faith traditions—Sunni Islam and African Catholicism—have been self-consciously selected for study; why the research is geographically located in Nairobi, Kenya; and why HIV and AIDS was chosen as the lens of comparative analysis. It then provides a brief overview of how adapting Fr. Agbonkhianmeghe E. Orobator's crisis-to-*kairos* framework, with which he explains the conceptual shift from a sociological issue as crisis to its theological response as *kairos*, is helpful in terms of presenting the research.[4] Finally, the chapter offers the chapter outlines for the rest of the manuscript and ends with a brief set of concluding remarks.

IN DEFENSE OF METHOD

The method adopted for this project involved six weeks of fieldwork during the summer of 2014 in Kenya's capital city of Nairobi to help fill in the interstices between anthropological, sociological, and ethnographic accounts provided by other leading academics in their respective fields.[5] It is additionally contingent on the fact that religious traditions in Kenya exhibit an openness and susceptibility to culture and context, as noted above. The practical openness to its social environment, then, affords this particular methodology a unique theological perspective which itself attempts to identify and analyze patterns of social behavior and religious organization. Though non-normative, this research proposes that certain observable phenomena can be compared between the two self-consciously selected religious groups in Nairobi, Kenya—Catholic on the one hand and Sunni Muslim on the other.

This research therefore suggests that among the Muslims and Catholics of Nairobi, religious practice can be located within a certain, specific, social context based on local human experience while also drawing on the larger identity of the worldwide population of religiously faithful through the transcendence of theology. For the purposes of this project, the methodology adopted in the form of interview data from twelve Muslim and Catholic leaders living in and around Nairobi does not assume exclusivity between the two elements of religious practice, the human and the divine. Rather, religious patterns of belief, action, and organization analyzed from the interview data reflect that this religious experience among Muslims and Catholics are influenced by scripture and revelation, as well as by society and culture.[6]

The next possibly evident methodological question is why conduct fieldwork in Nairobi, Kenya? In Nairobi, as in other parts of the world, the interaction between religious communities constitutes a rich source of material for any number of academic disciplines. From anthropology, to sociology, to history, to theology, those engaged in a critical survey of interreligious encounters must self-consciously acknowledge the social milieu within which such interactions occur. "The social sciences and humanities have long developed a strong interest in the Christian church and religion, greatly enhancing our understanding of how it functions and what it means in Africa," writes Fr. A. E. Orobator on the attention that the Catholic Church garners among other academic fields.[7]

Thus, when we look at the interplay between religions in Nairobi, it may be helpful to understand exactly which traditions we are exploring, as well as what we mean by religion in Kenya. In this East African country, roughly twice the land mass of the American state of Nevada, religious institutions operate as observable phenomena, even though they are continually changing to meet the needs of their respective congregations while coexisting with other recognizable social realities pursuing a "more or less clearly defined set of goals."[8]

Thus, speaking of one monolithic religious identity is largely impossible since it dismisses the unique particularity of lived religious practice, which itself informs religious experience and self-understanding. The Church and the mosque are not closed off from the rest of society. Rather, both are open and adaptive to the influence of the underlying society and culture.

On this topic, any religious movement engages two different yet complementary elements: on the one hand, religion exists in a specific social setting that fundamentally dictates how the religion operates in the human society; while, on the other hand, the religion itself contains a transcendent element that draws the faithful into something much larger and broader than the social setting within which they live and worship. And yet, even with this religious tether to both the mundane and the divine, due to numerous complex and interrelated factors, HIV continues to spread.[9]

Methodological Limitations

Such a proposed methodology cannot, by its very nature, explore every facet of religious experience since there are, indeed, many different forms of lived religious practice. Even between the two different religious traditions, at first glance it might seem as though the practical differences between Sunni Islam and Catholicism preclude any form of substantive comparison—even from a non-normative, descriptive standpoint. For this reason, the project and myself as the principal investigator must assume some methodological presuppositions. Since Islam and Catholicism in Kenya are lived traditions, there are then certain social issues and social facts that each group must consciously address. For example, it is a social fact that HIV infection rates in Kenya have leveled off during the past decade to 6.1 percent of the adult population.[10]

However, this still means that a significant portion of Kenyans are currently living with HIV and AIDS infection within Muslim and Christian communities.[11] Muslim and Catholic leaders in Nairobi are daily faced with the challenge of making sense of the epidemic, both practically and religiously. These officials find themselves between theology on the one hand and physiology on the other. Further, since an intersectional approach presumes any number of lenses for analyzing the subject at hand, the selection criteria for this project must be made quite specifically and with a specific purpose in mind. Because of this, the current research will be limited to theological responses of Muslim and Catholic religious leaders within their own communities, collected in the form of interview data through fieldwork. This obviously leaves certain questions unanswered, such as issues of ethnicity; the perspective of the laity; the overall voice of women; and topics related to Kenyan geography. Such are the shortcomings of the present endeavor, as it presents an incomplete picture of how Sunni Islam and African Catholicism are represented holistically, particularly as the aforementioned openness to context and culture creates a complex web of religious experience and identity.

This shortcoming, however, is not for lack of a specific focus. Rather, to reaffirm Claire Watkins's compelling observation regarding the organization of the Catholic Church, "Such is the complexity of the organizational life, in the Church as elsewhere, that to talk clearly and effectively means to talk about a limited and defined area, and not to deal in general and grand theory."[12]

Islam and Christianity in Kenya

The next methodological interrogative: Why study the Sunni Muslim and African Catholicism population of Nairobi? After all, these two religious groups do not constitute the largest populations of the religiously faithful throughout Nairobi—that honor belongs to the Protestant confessions which represent, according to some estimates, 47.4 percent of the Kenyan population.[13] Catholicism and Sunni Islam represent 23.3 percent and 11.1 percent, respectively, though these figures are open to creative interpretation since they have been collected by independent organizations, such as the CIA World Factbook, and not independently by the Kenyan government.[14] The reason this project self-consciously selected these religious groups is my familiarity with the doctrines and practice of both groups. As a Catholic raised in the Church and having attended Catholic parochial school for most of my life, the reason I selected Sunni Islam as the next interlocutor for discussion is my study and life among Muslim populations, both at home and abroad.

THE PRACTICAL AND THEOLOGICAL DIMENSIONS OF HIV AND AIDS IN KENYA

The AIDS epidemic in Kenya represents a distinct social issue since it affects both the Sunni Muslim and the African Catholic communities. From this, those persons religious living with the virus deal with the negative consequences of a lack of health care, ineffective education, and the stigma directed toward not only themselves but also their friends and family. The epidemic thus represents both a challenge and a *kairos* opportunity for religious leaders throughout Kenya in terms of society as well as in terms of theology. "It is so necessary for the religious leaders to come together to address the common problem that affects each and every one in the community," asserted one Muslim representative in Nairobi. "HIV does not discriminate based off anything. So it would be wise to come together as a community to fight the common problem for the community at large."[15] The unique social reality of the HIV and AIDS in Kenya represents not only a physiological challenge for health-care providers and medical workers, it also represents a collective challenge for both Muslim and Catholic leaders to come together in responding to the shared issue of HIV infection within their religious communities.

Such a proposed framework allows for a dual analysis of the contemporary, lived situation in Nairobi—one that illuminates some of the challenges and opportunities for those who are practically responding to the people negatively affected by the disease. From a religious perspective, people living with HIV and AIDS infection are often stigmatized and discriminated against by members of their own religious communities. This is not only unjust but it is also illegal according to the Constitution of Kenya, 2010.[16] The epidemic also lends itself to a positive analysis, that people from different faith traditions can and do come together in order to provide medical care and pastoral support for those individuals living with HIV and AIDS in both communities.

Because of this, both historically and even today, religious officials are faced with very real practical challenges in the areas of prevention, education, and destigmatization as this relates to HIV and AIDS in their own congregations. Yet, these same challenges when framed differently can actually be seen as opportunities for religious officials to come together, motivated by mercy, hospitality, and justice to provide pastoral care to those living with the disease irrespective of religious self-identification.

Thus, as a practical reality, HIV and AIDS affect both Muslim and Catholic communities in contemporary Kenya as both a challenge and an opportunity. Certain structural realities—among them poverty, access to health care, lack of education, and discrimination based on infection status—represent major obstacles and concerns for both faith communities.[17] The experience "of HIV is characterized by a struggle between truth and silence, and the need (for religious people, particularly) to find a language in which taboo issues may be discussed," asserts one Catholic voice, Gillian Paterson, in the discussion on HIV and AIDS structural causes. "The taboos that silence talk of sex and sexuality do not make people more moral: instead, they provide a safety zone for abuse by ensuring that the shock experienced when such things are spoken of relates less to the acts themselves than to the fact of their being mentioned at all."[18]

Or, put more bluntly from a Christian perspective, "*the body of Christ has AIDS*."[19] Given these observations, when religious institutions fail to address and speak openly about certain topics, such as transactional sex, intravenous drug use (IDU), condoms, gender roles, imprisonment, and homosexuality, they also fail the people most vulnerable to HIV and AIDS infection. As an epidemic, the disease in Kenya touches on many of the structural issues facing religious practice in Nairobi.

HIV and AIDS in Kenya

HIV infection rates have stabilized at 6.1 percent of the adult Kenyan population down from an all-time high of 10.5 percent in 1995–1996.[20] However, over 1.6 million Kenyans are currently living with the virus, many of who are drawn to urban centers such as Nairobi.[21] Undoubtedly, as has been made clear through the course of my interviews, the epidemic has negatively affected both Catholics and Sunni Muslims taking a tragic human toll. Consequently, living with the disease remains a reality for many faithful in both communities in Nairobi. HIV and AIDS, as will be explored elsewhere, presents a collective challenge and opportunity for both religions since members of their congregations are still susceptible to contracting the infection. "The crisis of AIDS, pernicious though it is," writes Orobator in Bénézet Bujo and Michael Czerny's edited volume, *AIDS in Africa: Theological Reflections*, "represents, in the terminology of Vatican II, 'signs of the times' and presents an opportune time or 'defining moment' (*kairos*) containing 'a clear and compelling call from God' to the Church"—to serve the poorest of the poor without judging.[22] While much of the focus of scholarly writing has been directed toward the Catholic Church and its response to AIDS in sub-Saharan Africa, Islam as a social reality that responds to its contextual environment is similarly addressing issues of health care, education, and stigma mitigation in a very practical sense. From the interviews conducted with both Catholic and Muslim leaders, it is clear from this research that HIV represents a modern crisis for both communities of faith since the disease carries with it both theological and biomedical considerations.

As a "sign of the times," the AIDS epidemic in Kenya is a unique entity forcing the religious faithful—specifically the religious leaders—to reconcile their divine mission within the mundane world. The persistence of HIV in Nairobi brings into focus some of the prominent social issues facing both Islam and Catholicism. The major line of inquiry undergirding this entire study lies in comparing how religious officials—priests and nuns, sheikhs and imams—far from standing in isolation from the lived reality of HIV and AIDS in their communities are actually responding to the epidemic through pastoral care, which itself entails theological and biological dimensions. As a matter of praxis, the pastoral care provided by persons religious in Kenya's capital city is performed for those with the infection who require care for both the body and soul. Pastoral care entails the health of the individual, both biological and religious notions pertaining to the holy and the mundane remain a central focus for comparison between Sunni Muslim and Catholic leaders.

One final note on the decision to select HIV and AIDS as the major theme for comparative analysis between Sunni Islam and African Catholicism in Nairobi and the religious significance of Islam and Catholicism in Kenya as recognizing that the epidemic continues to be a pervasive dilemma for both religions. As one Muslim official observed, "They say that Kenya is a religious community." He continued, "The majority of Kenyans—not all of them—but a majority of Kenyans . . . they believe in one religion or another. So they are either Christians, or Muslims, or Hindus, or whatever. But the majority of them, they believe in religion. And still, religious leaders are held in esteem."[23] As a very real crisis for these Muslim and Catholic leaders who are held in esteem by their congregations, AIDS is a disturbing reality since both religious traditions are open and deeply influenced by their social environments.

Given the significance of both Islam and Christianity for Kenya nationally, the epidemic in Nairobi raises major theological issues for both the Church and the mosque, with each group self-consciously striving to articulate in its activity. This observation does not realistically qualify whether the majority of Muslim and Catholic leaders are actually, adequately, or effectively coming to the aid of the infected and affected segments of their own population. The present research can offer insight into what these leaders say they are taking upon themselves to act as stewards of both the body and soul. This suggests that AIDS is a worrisome social reality for both faith traditions, one that represents an unavoidable dimension of religious experience in contemporary Kenya.

To conclude, this section has outlined, however briefly, the reasons for selecting HIV and AIDS as key social issues for analysis from the perspective of Sunni Islamic and African Catholic leadership. The main premise of this study rests on the assumption that the very nature of the epidemic in Nairobi represents a shared challenge for leaders from both faith traditions to address, assuage, and alleviate the lived experience of those members of their own congregations living with the disease—though this challenge is reframed as an opportunity for action in later chapters. Further, since HIV and AIDS draw our focus on both the practical and religious responses from both Islamic and Catholic institutions, the study proceeds with the belief that there are certain commonalities that can be compared—if not empirically, then at least descriptively—in their leaders' own words. To clarify the methodological approach adopted here, the rest of the chapter considers the use of field research as a method of data collection in assessing the lived Muslim and Catholic leadership's response to the epidemic from a theological perspective.

HIV and AIDS as both Crisis and *Kairos*

While the AIDS epidemic is, indeed, a challenge for the leaders of both religions, it also represents an opportunity—or to use the Catholic terminology, a *kairos* moment—for those working in disease prevention, education, and destigmatization. As a matter of conceptual clarification, I must admit that I employed, quite heavily at times, Fr. Orobator's distinction between HIV and AIDS as both a crisis and a *kairos*, which he addresses at length in his important 2005 work *From Crisis to Kairos: The Mission of the Church in the Time of HIV/AIDS, Refugees and Poverty*.

The reason this project adopts his binary classification is twofold: first, the disease has historically been a crisis for both faith communities, Muslim and Catholic alike. From the early 1980's in Kenya, the Church and the mosque were woefully ill-equipped to deal with the practical as well as the theological challenges of the epidemic. Since those dark days, both religions have made tremendous strides in the specific areas of prevention, education, and destigmatization after the leaders understood the presence of HIV as a *kairos* moment for God's decisive action. By recording and analyzing these religious officials' own words in the field, it is evident that—throughout Kenya, and in Nairobi specifically—the AIDS epidemic has shifted from crisis to *kairos*.

The second major reason this project uses Orobator's crisis-to-*kairos* framework is that it fundamentally deals with the methodological and conceptual crossroads between theology and praxis. As we will see later, AIDS in Kenya and throughout much of sub-Saharan Africa engages two worlds: first, crisis is a sociological distinction that has various dimensions—from human, to social, to economic, to cultural. Second, as a *kairos*, though, the epidemic has a distinct theological dimension, one which calls both Muslims and Catholics as communities of believers to come together to be a positive presence in the lives of those negatively affected by illness as the appointed time for God's presence.[24]

CHAPTER OUTLINES

Having treated many of the major methodological issues and questions pertaining to this research project, an overview of the chapters and their content is in order. In both chapters 1 and 2, the project adopts a structure that can be broken down into two complementary parts. The first major section offers an overview of religious responses to HIV and AIDS in Kenya from a historical vantage point, while in the second major section, the project considers the interview data collected to provide insight into official religious efforts toward the AIDS epidemic in Nairobi even today. Chapter 1 examines the Catholic tradition while chapter 2 examines the Islamic voice in responding to the disease. Also, as part of this structure, the analysis identifies three areas of strategic activity from within both religious communities—those of prevention, education, and destigmatization. The chapters also consider how these aims and efforts have changed and adapted since the early days of the disease by using Fr. Orobator's conceptual distinction of a movement from crisis to *kairos* to provide a descriptive account of how far each religion has come in dealing with those infected and those negatively affected by the AIDS epidemic in Nairobi.

Chapter 3 examines some major theological themes common to both Islam and Catholicism drawn out from the interviews presented in the preceding chapters. In this section, I posit that for each of the three identified areas of religious activity by Muslim and Catholic leaders there are certain theological traditions within each religion that correspond to these objectives. Namely, prevention efforts are motivated by mercy; education is motivated by the tradition of hospitality; and destigmatization efforts are motivated by justice, more specifically by social justice. The chapter makes use of scripture from both traditions to strengthen the connection between human activity and theological virtue common to both Islam and Catholicism.

In the concluding chapter 4, the project addresses one of the major lingering issues that remains from the research presented, that of sexuality and its impact on the ways in which Muslims and Catholics are responding to the HIV and AIDS epidemic in Nairobi. Within the overarching theme of sexuality, the chapter presents three specific areas that remain troublesome for both communities of faith, even with the advances made over the past thirty years. These areas—sexual intercourse, perceived gender roles, and condom use—represent areas of shared concern from both Muslim and Catholic leaders and shed some light on the possibility of further theological inquiry. After all, while there are doctrines for both Islam and Catholicism that dictate policy and activity, there are a broad range of opinions on the subject of sexuality, and this concluding chapter raises some of the major issues still facing those religious officials who respond to the disease and those negatively affected by HIV and AIDS infection on a daily basis.

CONCLUSION

It is my hope that this overall study provides a sufficiently theological account of how Muslim and Catholic leaders and their communities in Nairobi have provided care—and indeed are continuing to provide care—to those living with infection within their own congregations, and how the shared urgency of the epidemic has resulted in certain identifiable patterns of action and organization that are, at once, influenced by culture and theology. In this way, the project attempts to illuminate the crossroads between theology and lived religious experience that itself informs how religious communities self-consciously understand the present epidemic in Nairobi, from crisis to *kairos*.

NOTES

1. Jon Fuller, SJ and James Keenan, SJ, "Educating in a Time of HIV/AIDS: Learning from the Legacies of Human Rights, the Common Good, and the Works of Mercy," Julian Filochowski and Peter Stanford, eds. *Opening Up: Speaking Out in the Church* (London, UK: Darton, Longman, & Todd, 2005), 96–97. The opening quotation for this chapter comes from Muhammad ibn Abd 'Allah al-Khatb al-Tibriz, *Mishkat al-Masabih*, Vol. I, trans. James Robson (Islamabad, Pakistan: Orentalia Arts Ltd., 1999), 321.
2. See Victor Turner, *The Ritual Process: Structure and Anti-Structure* (Piscataway, NJ: Aldine Transaction, Reprint Edition, 1995), 4–6.
3. Jeffrey L. Tribble, "Ethnographic Research on African Pastoral Leadership and Congregations," in *Ethnography as Christian Theology and Ethics*, eds. Christian Scharen and Aana Marie Vigen (New York: Continuum International Publishing Group, 2011); Melissa Browning, "Theology and Morality on the Streets: An Examination of the Beliefs and Moral Formation of Street Children in Light of Christianity and African Traditional Religions," in *Ethnography as Christian Theology and Ethics*.
4. Agbonkhianmeghe E. Orobator, *From Crisis to Kairos*: *The Mission of the Church in the Time of HIV/AIDS, Refugees, and Poverty* (Nairobi, Kenya: Paulines Publications Africa, 2005).
5. The author here self-consciously acknowledges that one limitation of the present research undertaken for this book is that it is temporally localized to 2014. While there have been some positive advances in prevention, education, and destigmatization since then, much work remains from within both the Catholic and Islamic communities. Joint United Nations Programme on HIV/AIDS (UNAIDS), *UNAIDS Data 2017* (Geneva, Switzerland: UNAIDS Secretariat, 2017), 31.

6. Claire Watkins, "Organizing the People of God: Social-Science Theories of Organization in Ecclesiology," *Theological Studies* 52 (1991), 699.
7. Orobator, *From Crisis to Kairos*, 23.
8. Ibid.
9. Simon Ulrik Kragh, "The Anthropology of Nepotism: Social Distance and reciprocity in Organizations in Developing Countries," *International Journal of Cross Cultural Management* 12. 2 (August 2012): 247–65.
10. National AIDS Control Council (NACC), *Kenya AIDS Response Progress Report, 2014: Progress towards Zero* (Nairobi, Kenya: National AIDS Control Council of Kenya, 2014), 3.
11. Joint United Nations Programme on HIV/AIDS (UNAIDS), *Global Report: UNAIDS Report on the Global AIDS Epidemic 2013* (Geneva, Switzerland: UNAIDS Secretariat, 2013), A7.
12. Watkins, "Organizing the People of God," 709.
13. Central Intelligence Agency (CIA), "Africa—Kenya," in *The World Factbook 2003–14* (Washington DC: Central Intelligence Agency, 2013), 3.
14. Ibid.
15. Personal Interview—Nairobi, Kenya, 6.18.14.
16. National Council for Law Reporting, *The Constitution of Kenya [Kenya]* (Nairobi, Kenya: Kenyan National Legislative Bodies, 27 August 2010), §27.4.
17. Orobator, *From Crisis to Kairos*, 31.
18. Gillian Paterson, *Stigma in the Context of Development* (London, UK: Progressio, 2009), 10.
19. Donald E. Messer, *Breaking the Conspiracy of Silence: Christian Churches and the Global AIDS Crisis* (Minneapolis, MN: Fortress Press, 2004), 19.
20. NACC, *Kenya AIDS Response Progress Report, 2014*, 3.
21. UNAIDS, *Global Report,* A7.
22. Agbonkhianmeghe E. Orobator, "When AIDS Comes to Church" in *AIDS in Africa: Theological Reflections*, eds. Bénézet Bujo and Michael Czerny (Nairobi, Kenya: Paulines Publications Africa, 2007), 128.
23. Personal Interview—Nairobi, Kenya, 6.12.14.
24. Orobator, "When AIDS Comes to Church," 128.

Chapter One

"I was sick and you took care of me"

Catholic Responses to HIV and AIDS in Nairobi, Kenya

INTRODUCTION AND PLAN FOR THE CHAPTER

One of the largest religious traditions in Kenya, Catholicism has a long history in Eastern Africa.[1] From colonization to the twenty-first century, the Catholic Church both institutionally and practically has a profound impact in determining how Kenya's Catholic population understands their religious identity. This is particularly true in the capital city of Nairobi where traditional Catholic values interface with modernity, urbanity, and religious pluralism. Through its activities in education, health care, and grassroots advocacy, the Church has tremendous authority over how Kenyan Catholics practice their faith. As this relates to HIV and AIDS, the Catholic Church and specifically Catholic leaders are active in three major strategic areas of interest: prevention and health care, education, and destigmatization

This chapter begins with an overview of the Catholic Church's historical development in Eastern Africa, including a brief discussion of the interaction and exchange of religious views between Catholicism and traditional African religion. The chapter then proposes a framework for analyzing the three areas of church activity in responding to HIV and AIDS in Nairobi as a movement from crisis to *kairos* as adapted from the work of Fr. A. E. Orobator.[2] The latter half of the chapter considers, in the very words of Catholic officials, how the Church has responded to the AIDS epidemic in Nairobi in each of the three identified areas as a shift from the sociological category of crisis to the theological category of *kairos*.[3] From this crisis-to-*kairos* distinction the research focuses on the practical response of Catholic leaders and how these officials live their faith in the age of this epidemic. This general framework will also be employed and adapted for the subsequent chapter which considers the Sunni Muslim response to HIV and AIDS in Nairobi.

COLONIALISM, TRADITIONAL AFRICAN RELIGION, AND THE CATHOLIC CHURCH

Catholicism has long been a major influence in the religiously pluralistic milieu of Kenya. The Portuguese introduced Catholicism to East Africa in 1498 through mission work and the establishment of Catholic charities, school, and hospitals. The Church was able to gain adherents through conversions, both voluntary and forced.[4] Historically, Catholic leaders initially faced the challenge as to what extent foundational teachings could be synthesized with traditional African religions. "In a sense, the religious practice—the indigenous religious practice—serves as a kind of substratum on which Christianity and Islam, sit; they sit on this base," in the words of one Catholic leader living in Nairobi. "So that even if people become Muslims or Christians, that core is still very active, or rather can be activated especially at times of crisis. So it's a reality in people's lives that I would certainly not deny. It is present."[5]

This self-conscious assessment of the relationship between Catholicism and traditional African religion is compelling. Early missionaries were forced to negotiate with existing religious and cultural structures in order to gain converts.[6] This has historically led to the creation of a unique understanding of the Catholic Church in Eastern Africa and particularly in Nairobi where the rich mixture of ethnicity, culture, and language has allowed a specifically Kenyan Catholicism to develop and blossom.

Not long after spreading from the Swahili coastal region along the Indian Ocean in the mid- to late-sixteenth century, Catholic missionaries and converts began founding schools and hospitals in order to provide tangible resources to the new Catholics, maintaining a positive presence in the communities within which their religion was practiced.[7] Thus, the Church established the social structures providing both Catholics and non-Catholics with certain basic needs—such as education and health care—which constitute the very basis of Western concepts of social welfare.[8] The result of the rapid expansion of this social welfare and the lasting presence of both doctor and educator helps explain the current estimates suggesting the current population of Catholics in Kenya at 23.3 percent of the overall Kenyan population.[9]

Catholicism in Kenya is a prominent religious voice in society. Studies show that about 30 percent of all health care—nearly one out of three hospital beds throughout Kenya—are run by the Catholic Church or by Catholic-affiliated charities and organizations.[10] It is evident that the Church plays an important role and maintains an active presence in the field of HIV and AIDS care, prevention, and treatment. Because of its long history in East Africa, in addition to its selfless work in charity, education, and health care, the Catholic Church is uniquely suited to address issues of both a spiritual and corporeal nature.

Advancing the need for an ethic based in care and compassion that acknowledges and attempts to assuage human suffering as a primary motivation, far from attempting to isolate each constituent element of the Church response to the AIDS epidemic—that is, the human and the divine—each dimension cannot fully be experienced or understood without explicitly acknowledging the other. Noted Catholic ethicist, Margaret A. Farley, writes on compassion, "because compassion involves a beholding of the value of others and a suffering with them in their need, it opens reality to the beholder; it offers a way of "seeing" that evokes a moral response."[11] This need, of course, involves both physical and spiritual responses. That the Catholic Church inhabits both realms is singularly notable, making it an inviting topic for studying how church leadership is practically responding to HIV and AIDS in Kenya. This is further supported by its location geographically, as sub-Saharan Africa has been inordinately affected by the pandemic, with Eastern Africa bearing much of this tragic statistic.[12]

In Kenya, even with government sanctioned and designed programs focusing on education and prevention, the epidemic remains a lived reality for over 1.6 million Kenyans, with young adults and women representing the majority of this statistic.[13] With such a disproportionate number of affected and infected individuals compared to the West, the Catholic Church in Kenya is actively called to address the issue, chiefly in the areas of prevention and health care, education, and stigma mitigation.

"WHO DO THE CROWDS SAY THAT I AM?" AFRICAN CATHOLICS ON HIV AND AIDS

From a Catholic perspective, the AIDS epidemic in Kenya's capital and most populous city raises certain theological and ethical questions that concern the human person.[14] Priests and women religious throughout the country have been and are continually charged with providing resources for both the spirit and the temporal needs of their congregations. A pivotal aspect of this religious response in Kenya then involves those Catholic religious figures working in the field of disease prevention, education, and stigma reduction. By considering the lived religious response to HIV and AIDS in Kenya, Roman Catholic leaders living in Nairobi can bring about the preferential and effective attention to the dignity, needs, and rights of those living with disease.

While this book explores the voice of actual Kenyan theologians on the topics of HIV and AIDS prevention, education, and destigmatization,

Nairobi has no lack of both official and popular opinion on the country's epidemic, meaning the various religious traditions display their own internal and external views on how to address those negatively affected by the virus.[15] Therefore, it may be helpful here to offer an overview of several Kenyan theologians on the topic of HIV and AIDS.

First, in general terms, addressing a contextualized approach to Christian theology in an African setting, noted Catholic theologian Laurenti Magesa, professor of ethics at Hekima University in Nairobi writes, "The African worldview is spiritual but deeply life-oriented in practice. Seemingly 'ordinary' behavior is invariable laden with mystical (spiritual) meaning whose import must be constantly interpreted in as much as it transcends conventional appearances." He continues, "From this perspective, the ultimate meaning of any thought, act, or word must be sought in its relationship to, and effects on, human existence: whether it promotes the good life that is the door to human transcendent existence."[16]

In this broad African worldview, the existence of HIV and AIDS is a severe impediment for those who continue to strive for the good life, both personally and communally, while moralistic views directed toward those who have contracted the human immunodeficiency virus detract from the longevity of the overall health of the community. Magesa concludes on the African response to HIV and AIDS, "What is needed is an approach that can transform Africa's own symbolism, imagery and linguistic frames of reference towards abundant life. What are required are perceptions that take into account what this central value entails in the current context of HIV and AIDS." Further, he proposes that "three major, interrelated components emerge from within African culture itself as sources of transforming action: namely, solidarity, compassion, and responsibility—all of them intrinsic dimensions to African community."[17]

An interesting parallel, Magesa identifies three salient values to the African community and its approach to HIV and AIDS not dissimilar to the ones analyzed in this work. These three components—solidarity, compassion, and responsibility—constitute the basis for an African theology directed toward those living with illness, particularly in the case of HIV and AIDS in Kenya. While not exclusive to Catholicism, these theological elements concern the cultural and social context of all who provide care to those negatively affected by the epidemic in Nairobi.

More specifically, Kenyan Catholic theologian Festo Mkenda, SJ, reflects on the image of community and the African family when he writes, "The African women and the African family stand out as two pillars without which society should have collapsed under the AIDS crisis."[18] As with Laurenti Magesa, the salient elements of community and solidarity stand out as important virtues in addressing HIV and AIDS in an African setting as issues of gender roles and sexuality come to play a huge part in how African societies address the AIDS epidemic in Kenya. Acknowledging the communal nature of African society, Mkenda also notes, "Like the woman, the African extended family absorbed the heaviest shocks of AIDS," concluding, "the divine persons see opportunities for positive action where humans might see none. Learning from them, we might identify similar opportunities even in the cinders left by the regretted virus and disease."[19] Undoubtedly, theology and modernity maintain a tense relationship in Nairobi—a topic explored elsewhere in this book—and yet those most vulnerable, such as women, children, and the elderly bear much of the burden of the AIDS epidemic, not only in Kenya, but also throughout the world. The vulnerability of these demographics is equally telling and equally trying, in that those most in need of social justice represent those who are often overlooked by other segments of society.

To this end, and more specifically considering the voice of women in the Kenyan Catholic discourse surrounding HIV and AIDS, sexuality and gender dynamics remain important dimensions of the epidemic in Kenya. And yet, where the various religions of Nairobi—in this particular section, Kenya Catholic theologians—look to the place of women as integral to community, certain challenges remain in responding to the AIDS epidemic in Eastern Africa. One Kenyan female theologian, Teresia Mbari Hinga, identifies several theological hurdles the Church faces in moving forward to address the AIDS epidemic in Kenya. A member of the Circle of Concerned African Women Theologians (CCAWT, also "the Circle"), she observes certain entrenched theological practices—such as marriage—reinforce patriarchy within the Catholic Church.[20]

What is needed, in her opinion, is a theology of equality that affirms the inherent dignity of women in African society in its approach to AIDS, thereby requiring a theological response that places women and those most vulnerable at the center of Catholic efforts in education, prevention, and destigmatization. "One of the most enduring crises that the world has faced in the last three decades and more is the HIV and AIDS crisis. The crisis has been exacerbated by a variety of issues, including stigma against the African continent itself as well as against people living with HIV," she writes.[21] Further, as a member of the CCAWT, Hinga notes that the members of the Circle "have proposed, and indeed practice, alternative ways of wielding power and authority. De jure, if not entirely de facto, the ideal for them is to nurture and implement the ideas of 'power with' and 'power for' others rather than 'power over.' "[22] This spotlight on notions of gender in facing the reality of HIV and AIDS in Kenya is particularly relevant to this work since women are at once actively engaged in advocacy in areas where women are disproportionately affected by the epidemic in Kenya.[23]

These deeply theological terms—society, equality, community, compassion, solidarity, dignity, and responsibility—manifest a uniquely African yet universally human approach to combatting the spread of HIV and AIDS in Kenya. And where these Catholic theologian, self-consciously and self-reflexively, try to make sense of the ravages of AIDS in their own communities, relying on an African purview, it is quite clear that no quick fix is readily available. "Clearly," Hinga writes, "there is work to be done in search for an AIDS-free world."[24] Particularly as this relates to notions of gender and sexuality to be explored later in this book, as we consider the contributions of these Kenyan theologians, each raises a new vantage point with which we can consider the AIDS epidemic in Kenya. Yet, regarding the AIDS pandemic in sub-Saharan Africa, "we might discover that we still have a great deal to learn."[25]

When applied to the worldwide reality of HIV and AIDS, those living with any form of disease or illness can be treated partly in terms of biomedicine and partly in terms of faith. The rest of this initial chapter proceeds in this way—prevention, education, and destigmatization. After an initial examination of church policy in Kenya, the section then reviews the binary distinction of HIV and AIDS in sub-Saharan Africa as a sociological crisis and a theological *kairos*. With the structure developed, the subsequent section applies the crisis/*kairos* characterization to prevention, education, and stigma mitigation as expressed by actual Catholic leaders living among and facing daily the challenge and opportunity of HIV and AIDS within the Catholic community of Nairobi.

Prevention and Health Care

General issues of prevention and health care remain one of the largest practical challenges facing religious leaders engaged in public health initiatives in Nairobi. "Prevention of HIV," writes the Kenyan Episcopal Conference (KEC), "is based on open communication, better understanding, firm values and avoidance of high risk behavior."[26] This assessment by the church leadership in Kenya calls attention to two competing spheres of influence in HIV prevention throughout the country. First, it acknowledges that there is the need for a theological grounding in combatting disease transmission, namely "firm values" and "better understanding." Second, and equally important, the KEC acknowledges that humans by their very nature are likely to engage in human behavior and be attracted to human temptation. Faithful Catholics are thus called to avoid such "high risk behavior."

The bishops of Kenya explicitly set out strategic objectives regarding prevention initiatives—from blood safety, to mother-to-child transmission (MTCT), to voluntary counseling and testing (VCT)—since one of the most formidable issues of HIV prevention is access to health care. "We urge the members of the Church in our countries, laity and clergy, cooperating where possible with already existing organization to search for the most effective means of help," the bishops of the KEC entreat, "and we ask our bishops to give their active support to this work of Christ: for it is His Body which has AIDS."[27] The imagery employed by the Catholic bishops of Kenya highlights some of the pressing and very real issues facing the Church in Kenya. In terms of prevention and health care, the Roman Catholic Church inhabits a distinct position of treating both spiritually and physically those living with the disease. Stated differently, "the Church cares pastorally and often medically for the sick, advocating their access to treatment. A large proportion of healthcare and medical treatment is already offered by Catholic clinics, hospitals, parishes and other institutions, and we renew our commitment to make as many resources available as possible," the bishops of the Kenyan Episcopal Conference continue. "But let everything be done, not only with efficiency and professional competence, but also with the hands and mind and heart of Jesus—not just excellent but clearly Christian."[28]

This concluding addendum that the Church response in Kenya should be "excellent" and "clearly Christian" once again affirms the Catholic mandate that engages the dual identity of the Church as a religious and social institution. Catholic leaders are working to theologically attend to the physiological and social dimensions of being human and so this is a challenging and remarkable opportunity. The health of the Church is directly related to the health of the community as both in many ways are interrelated. Regarding the communal health of the entire population of Kenyan Catholics, the Kenyan bishops implore, "Please give us the support of our faith, give us the guidance and orientation of our Church's teaching, as we deal with the questions, doubts, fears and dilemmas of Kenyans, all of us burdened in one way or another by HIV and AIDS."[29] Just as the condition of community health is contingent on the health of each individual, Catholic strategic goals in prevention, education, and destigmatization are likewise interconnected and interdependent on each other. Since one major element of prevention involves education, the next section considers some of the initiatives begun by the Catholic Church for HIV and AIDS education in Nairobi.

HIV and AIDS Education

"I think—I am more and more convinced that my conversations with the African Bishops—that the basic question, if we want to move ahead in this field [of HIV and AIDS] is about education, training," reflects Pope Benedict XVI. "Progress becomes true progress only if it serves the human person and if the human grows, not in terms of technical power alone, but in moral capacity too."[30] The pope's prescient account of the aims of education demands the development and formation of the whole human person—both body and soul—which includes the moral and mental faculties of the human mind as well. For this reason, education is fundamentally important for the

Catholic Church and its response to AIDS in Kenya, since it sets the vocabulary and tone of the agenda.

Citing the need for religious educational resources for all Kenyans, the bishops of the KEC spell out their strategic objectives as follows:

> The Church in Kenya will strive to increase general capacity for HIV prevention through formation for responsible and respectful behavior as well [as] education about HIV, AIDS and sexuality, based on full, accurate and scientific information. Information will be tailored to reach and suit different audiences such as children, youth, females and adults in general.

The bishops continue:

> In order to diminish inequalities and abuse which fuel the spread of HIV, the Church will promote education of women, their empowerment and leadership. Concomitantly, the Church will impart life skills to men, women, children and youth, enabling them to make informed and responsible decisions.[31]

That the KEC self-consciously emphasizes the dimension of gender and sexuality in its educational objectives is worth examining, since the KEC as a constituent body is solely comprised of men. The Catholic Church, as a patriarchal, education-providing institution that specifically focuses on the empowerment of youth and females, highlights the multifaceted and interdisciplinary nature of the lived religious response to HIV and AIDS in Nairobi. Taking this reflexive inventory of areas of education that most need clarification or improvement, the bishops seem to endorse a refining of educational endeavors by the Church since education can be transformative and empowering for "children, youth, females, and adults in general." "Using appropriate media channels," the Kenyan bishops propose, "the Church will educate about HIV prevention, exercise its leading role in stigma reduction, and endorse positive, responsible behavior in line with the Church's moral values like respect for others, self-respect, and protection of life and the promotion of family."[32]

Not only does the Church enunciate its authority as an educational leader in this excerpt, but it also draws into focus the diverse and interrelated elements of its educational objectives—chief among them the other two areas of analysis proposed at the outset of this chapter, "HIV prevention" and "stigma reduction." In other words, "alongside pastoral ministry, medical care, and the practice of compassion and advocacy, the Church also keeps a firm place for personal *morality*, social *ethics*, and education for *prevention*."[33] Morality, ethics, and prevention might then be best understood as bearing some striking similarity, at least conceptually from the Catholic perspective. In many ways, then, education, prevention, and destigmatization inhabit much of the same theoretical space, both theologically and practically. The next section now considers programs for fighting stigma as one of the strategic aims of the KEC and for the entire Catholic Church in Kenya.

Stigma Mitigation and the Catholic Church

Stigma reduction is perhaps the most troubling of the three areas of church advocacy and response as it aims to fundamentally change the way people understand the etiology of HIV infection as well as its modes of transmission. In the words of one prominent Catholic leader, Fr. Michael Czerny, SJ, who has worked in the field of HIV and AIDS prevention for over the past twenty years, "Stigma is a mark, a sign, a label. It refers to negatively perceived characteristics which set individuals or groups apart from the normal social order. If someone near us or known to us were to become HIV+, would we tend 'for good reasons' to discriminate, exclude and stigmatize?" Fr. Czerny concludes, "Stigma is part of that common fabric of classification and rules which we call culture, and because it is interpersonal and unspoken, it commands huge power."[34]

When this stigma is directed toward the AIDS epidemic in Kenya, the result is even more challenging since popular perceptions regarding transmission generally involve topics of sexuality. In setting the tone of the discussion, the bishops of Kenya recognize this apparent tension between HIV infection and sexuality when they write, "Among the many complex factors involved, that of *sexuality* seems to be the most difficult to talk about."[35] As an agent of change and evangelization, the Catholic Church in Kenya positions itself as an important force in combatting stigma from a theological view to empower those living with infection. "We are particularly distressed by the stigma attached to people living with AIDS and their families," the Kenyan bishops continue. "We call upon all Christians to overcome any prejudice they feel toward any AIDS victims. Even when contracted through immoral behavior—and we know it can be contracted through other ways—AIDS as a disease is not different from cancer and malaria."[36]

This last assertion on immorality serves to address much of the apprehension that Catholic leaders exhibit in speaking about stigma, as HIV and AIDS infection have often and historically been associated with individuals who had gone against the social or moral order. Specifically, as this relates to stigma reduction, the Church does acknowledge that there are those among its ranks for whom "the possibility of infection was due to behavior which many see as shameful."[37] The unintended consequence of this line of thinking involves a moralistic reading of the situation and in many ways seeks to blame the individual for contracting the disease. As an agent of empowerment and acceptance, the Catholic Church in Kenya can seek to diminish the risk of stigma by affirming the inherent dignity of the person living with infection, as well as helping their families by reinforcing the belief that "No one on earth has access to another's conscience, and no one can judge whether or not an individual has sinned, only the person in the presence of God."[38] Thus, by teaching about the disease and its transmission with "warmth, clarity, and courage" church officials and clergy can begin to bring about a change in understanding stigma and AIDS infection.[39]

According to the bishops, stigma reduction is at the forefront of the national campaign and among the strategic aims of the Conference:

> Stigma and discrimination make the general public afraid, with individuals afraid to find out their HIV status, or to seek care and support, or to do anything which might manifest their HIV-positive status. To deal with this cultural problem, the Church will use its well-established structures and systems (including homilies, media, and schools) to educate communities about HIV and AIDS and counteract stigma and discrimination.[40]

While the Church in this instance attributes stigma and discrimination as a "cultural problem," there are decidedly theological and religious dimensions to the problem of stigma. This is why, as a divine mandate, church leaders facing the negative impact of stigma in their own religious communities are called to imitate Jesus Christ. "[T]he Church typically works, humanely, materially, and spiritually, to bring consolation to orphans, widowers and widows, grandparents and the whole families as well as to vulnerable children and women whose lives have been wrecked as the result of the disease," writes Fr. Czerny. "To include the excluded, in other words, and to embrace and touch the stigmatized."[41] The essential quality of the Church strategy for addressing issues associated with HIV and AIDS in Kenya according to Fr. Czerny—that of the inherent dignity of those living within disease. As a matter concerned with Catholic social teaching, the dignity of those living with disease must never be diminished due to sickness and suffering, and must take part in the common good of society. Stigma and discrimination are thus anathema to Catholic social teaching. The Catholic Church is called to participate in the national response to HIV and AIDS by combatting stigma in its own community of believers.

The areas of Roman Catholic activity in Nairobi just examined—prevention, education, and destigmatization—while not a comprehensive list of overall church strategies do represent three explicit and deeply interrelated responses to those negatively affected by the AIDS epidemic in Kenya. Elements of prevention overlap with education which are informed by an attention to stigma mitigation efforts. Nevertheless, within each of these fields, this research discerns a conceptual dichotomy for how the disease was historically understood and addressed in a practical sense. Stated differently, whereas prevention, education, and destigmatization present the Church in Kenya with an opportunity to come to the aid—religiously and practically—for those living with HIV and AIDS infection, these objectives also constitute a very real challenge for Catholicism since religious leaders are called to change dominant views associated with the disease. For this reason, the next section describes Fr. A. E. Orobator's distinction of the epidemic as both a crisis and a *kairos* allowing for both a social and theological engagement with the disease and its effect on the people of Kenya.

THE AIDS EPIDEMIC: CRISIS AND *KAIROS*

A major figure in the field of Catholic advocacy on HIV and AIDS in Nairobi, Fr. Orobator in his work *From Crisis to Kairos*, refers to the epidemic in sub-Saharan Africa as both a crisis and a *kairos* or the appointed time for God's presence. This distinction is useful for the present study since, as previously noted, the classification of crisis represents a social reality where the classification of *kairos* represents a theological reality:

> Considered as a crisis, HIV and AIDS is a complex issue, incorporating many dimensions: social, medical, political, cultural, economic, religious, ethical and anthropological. There is a dynamic connection between *crisis* and *kairos*. Under the sociological category of *crisis*, HIV and AIDS demarcates a broad field of activity calling for the discernment, decision, judgment and participation of all sectors of society. Under the theological mode of *kairos*, it creates a platform on which the Church deploys its evangelizing and salvific mission in society as "a sacrament, a sign and instrument" of a compassionate God "who continually creates, redeems, and fulfills" humanity.[42]

This dichotomy between crisis and *kairos* illuminates the often tense relationship between society and theology. In referencing to the Catholic Church as both universal and particular, local and global, he rightly states that, "As the body of Christ, the Church is both an incarnate local community of faith and a universal sacrament of communion with God."[43] Since the Church is able to bridge the seemingly vast divide between the human and the divine worlds, the AIDS epidemic in Kenya represents a distinctive challenge for religious leaders.

First, the challenge can be formulated in negative terms since, in the areas of prevention, education, and destigmatization, the Church has historically been guilty of disseminating false notions of disease transmission, a moralistic reading of sexuality, and an outright condemnation and discrimination of people and the families of people living with the virus.[44] Lamentably, some church leaders have even encouraged negative trends like stigmatization and moral judgmentalism. "The priest has a lot and does say a lot about HIV and AIDS," said one priest living and serving the Catholic community of Nairobi. "The problem though is a question of knowledge, lack of knowledge—just like the rest of society. Sometimes I feel I have seen situations where it is very clear that the priests are poorly informed about HIV and AIDS—I mean, all aspects of it."[45]

With such a lack of knowledge to address the pressing concerns related to HIV and AIDS and its transmission, it is evident that the Catholic Church as a religious institution faces some very problematic hurdles to overcome, both internally and conceptually, with regard to the epidemic in Kenya. Instead of recriminations and moral judgment, "People with AIDS and their families should be able to count on the community of faith as a lasting source of support and care."[46]

This then brings us to the second dimension of the AIDS crisis in Kenya, the challenge to the Church in positive terms. The Catholic Church represents a community of faith, adequately suited to revolutionize human thought and action. When posed this way, the epidemic as *kairos* "implies that God dwells in the reality under consideration, which presence stimulates a new understanding of and a positive individual and collective response to that reality. When applied to the crisis of AIDS, one could argue that it represents a *kairos* for the Church."[47] With a radical reinterpretation of the disease, the Church calls its leadership to engage the present epidemic as agents of empowerment, evangelization, and change. After all, it is through reformulating the challenge of HIV and AIDS in positive terms that church officials must understand the disease as a "pathology of the spirit" to use Pope John Paul II's theological terminology, which also includes understanding the disease in human terms, with human faces to engage in a response to the epidemic that incorporates realistic human behavior.[48]

In recognizing the dual identity of HIV from a religious perspective in Kenya, justice calls for the Catholic Church to move beyond focusing on the negative aspects of the epidemic and instead call for an emphasis on the transformative and salvific nature of the Church as it lives and serves throughout Kenya. According to Orobator, it is only through a paradigm shift from darkness to light that the Church will act as the sign and instrument of a compassionate God that redeems and perfects humanity even in the face of intense human suffering. As a community of believers, the Church defines and fulfills its mission within the context of society, which implies ethics, cultural sensitivities, and the acknowledgment that this relationship reflects certain social and historical realities.

Because the Church as a theological institution operates in the human world, "Any theology of AIDS worthy of the name must be earthed in a living experience of HIV and AIDS."[49] The remainder of this chapter offers detailed accounts and analyses of Catholic religious leaders living, teaching, and working in Nairobi, Kenya, in their own words from interview data. However, a note on method is in order.

Prevention as Crisis

"No, no. HIV/AIDS has not gone away. It's there. We are still being infected, yes. I mean there have been significant strides in, for example, in preventing mother-to-child transmission, but the general problem remains that people are still being infected, and HIV and AIDS has no cure. We now deal with it as if it's not a problem."[50] This observation made by a prominent Catholic priest working in the field of HIV and AIDS education and research calls attention to the lack of contemporary concern regarding HIV and AIDS infection in Kenya's national discourse. Perhaps overshadowing the efforts of many community-based organizations (CBO), faith-based organizations (FBO), and non-governmental organizations (NGO), is this mistaken conception that the municipal disease prevention efforts and the relative accessibility of anti-retroviral therapy (ART) and voluntary counseling and testing (VCT) centers has given the public a false calm that the disease is no longer a threat.

It is precisely because of this view that infection rates have risen, even as Catholic-based organizations, along with secular programs like the President's Emergency Program for AIDS Relief (PEPFAR) and the Clinton Foundation, have reduced international aid.[51] Many of the priests, officials, and educators interviewed for this project looked to the historical roots of the disease as the logical starting point for the conversation. With regard to prevention in the 1980s, the early stages of the epidemic, the priest remarked:

> I think it's gone through phases especially in Kenya here. Again, the typical issues of denial were very much part of the initial response. But in the 1990s, the government set up the National AIDS Commission and really invested heavily—again partly because HIV/AIDS attracted a lot of international attention so we wouldn't be isolated—invested heavily in HIV/AIDS prevention and care—and also education, such that today I think in Kenya as well as the rest of the region, awareness is quite high. You know, HIV/AIDS people compared to other countries such as in Asia, for example, its awareness of HIV and AIDS is very very high. And that's due partly to the investment of the 1990s.[52]

While the initial impact of the disease on the Kenyan population demanded positive, practical results, as with any national emergency, the funding as well as international exposure declined, such that while the average Kenyan was well-versed in the complex language of biomedicines—AZT, ART, VCT, PLWHA, and so on—this education did little to mitigate the risk of people contracting the disease as other-izing behavior which did not take seriously the threat of contracting infection. The priest continued:

> But since the 2000's, I would say things have settled a bit because HIV/AIDS is not considered as a crisis that it was in the 80's and 90's. So you don't hear

> much being said about it. That same kind of consistent response by the government is certainly not there anymore, in the sense that HIV/AIDS is being mainstreamed, as in to general public health issues such that it doesn't enjoy that status of exceptionality that generated a lot of responses and resources, say in the past decades. So in a sense, I would say that it is regrettable because it does take away that sense of urgency. It does create the impression that the problem is no longer there. Which can then begin to drive up infection rates again and can lead to complacency. I think we have sort of been very complacent.[53]

Terms such as "denial" and "complacency" serve to offer insight into the self-critical analysis of the early days of the epidemic in Kenya, with religious leaders and governmental representatives trying to spearhead prevention initiatives to bring the disease into the national spotlight. However, again, when the disease was first officially detected and diagnosed in 1984 in Kenya, there were no real prevention programs in place to deal with those living with or personally affected by the disease.[54]

On the topic of denial, another Catholic official, leading prevention efforts in a Catholic Church affiliated home for AIDS orphans said:

> Well first of all, of course, there was denial. When the first case was identified in 85, we don't have HIV. And actually it was only when the then president, President Daniel Arap Moi, declared HIV a national catastrophe . . . in 99. Then the secrecy started to ease. Before that, there was dreadful secrecy about it, and the whole experience of HIV was the same experience as in the early 80's in USA. And people would present themselves emaciated, suffering from opportunistic infections—you know, Kaposi's Sarcoma. You see that, the wounds on the legs, etcetera. And loss of weight. So that was the experience of HIV.[55]

This observation paints a grim picture of the early days of HIV prevention efforts. It highlights certain failings by the Kenyan government as well as religious misunderstandings of the disease, specifically drawing the link between suffering and silence.[56]

While the subject offered critical insight into the moralistic reading of disease transmission in the early days of the epidemic in Nairobi. Many were infected with HIV due to unscreened blood transfusions as well as MTCT. Interestingly, moral judgment was also directed to the families of those living with infection who were similarly perceived with negative connotations. "And if your family—if one of your family had it—then you kept it secret as much as possible. You hid it, you kept it very quiet," stated the subject. "But from 1999 when it became much more open, then the response to [the disease] would have also. You see, in the developing world we're cash-strapped in the whole issue of HIV. So it's been a slow painful journey trying to answer to the needs of persons with HIV."[57]

Thus, where clergy initially sought to provide remedies for the negative aspects of the epidemic—namely denial, silence, secrecy—there exists some obvious methodological overlap between the religious and the secular governmental response. Because of this overlap, religious leaders were forced to acquaint themselves with the complex political mechanisms of international aid and familiarize themselves with the sophisticated language of medical treatment, health care, and prevention. "When PEPFAR came in, we were one of the first 16 countries that the US government identified back in 2003. That was tremendous," this member of the clergy asserted, addressing the conceptual crisis of HIV prevention. "We got access. But . . . it's been a huge struggle for the government because of the financial commitment since then."[58]

Yet with this promise of international support to identify and establish prevention programs in Nairobi there also arose the need to articulate the relationship between Catholic charities and exactly what these prevention efforts looked like for the international donors. "There is no way that we're in a position to buy the anti-retroviral medication at the prices at which it is available in the developed world. The very wealthy, maybe not even the top 10 percent, the top 6 percent percentage could afford to pay for the drugs," remarked the subject. "But the vast majority—99 percent can't afford the drugs. So we're dependent on getting the drugs through PEPFAR and the other organizations."[59]

This agreement—that PEPFAR and other international aid organizations would provide treatment for people living with HIV and AIDS (PLWHA) through Catholic charities, CBO's, and FBO's—forced Catholics working in the field of disease prevention to take account and understand the dynamics of this financial arrangement. Indeed, accepting such charity fundamentally changed the nature of the relationship between the Church and foreign donors. This became especially true when these aid organizations began to reduce funding for HIV and AIDS prevention, as PEPFAR did throughout the past decade. The religious mandate to provide care for those living with infection has thus been problematized by Catholic-affiliated health-care providers who have relied on these resources as a primary source of funding.

"The government has been challenged by PEPFAR in later years to take on the HIV issue more. And of course PEPFAR is not right-sizing Kenya, they've started to reduce the funding," confirmed the subject, even in relation to AIDS orphanages in Nairobi. "This happened for us as well, we call it 'country operation program.' October 2013 to the end of September 2014, we've had a cut of the PEPFAR funds, and we'll have a bigger cut next year. In other words, the US is challenging Kenya to really put more of the budget into HIV care and treatment."[60]

These financial concerns are worth noting, since many FBO's, orphanages, hospitals, and prevention initiatives rely on funds from external, secular, international organizations for their budgets. And, as a matter of externality, those people living with or personally affected by the epidemic are the ones who feel the very real impact of this reduction in funding. However, particularly in the field of prevention, what began as a state of crisis, or "national catastrophe" named by then Kenyan president, Daniel Arap Moi, in 1999, certain positive trends began to emerge, though partially and slowly. Even with a reduction in funding for Catholic institutions serving the population of Nairobi living with HIV and AIDS, the subject concludes, "The other trend is—and this is healthy—that, whereas in the beginning and right up to the present time, the services for HIV were separate from the ordinary medical services. They're trying now to integrate the services for HIV into the ordinary medical services. So this also reduces the discrimination side of the care and treatment."[61]

While HIV services are being subsumed by the national Kenyan general medical services prompted by the ratification of the Constitution of Kenya in 2010, budgetary constraints can be felt in many of the prevention efforts organized and led by members of the Catholic leadership.[62] Because these programs are so reliant on foreign donors, the issue of actually funding certain prevention efforts is at the forefront of Catholic discourse. "I know it's a budget issue, it's the willingness. More can be done. More can be done, I think that we always worry that a lot of the HIV budget is donor funded. And there's always this issue one day when the money freezes up," one Catholic interlocutor working in higher education remarked, "What will you do? You have thousands of people on ART's. You have orphans. So I think the government needs to own the project—they are trying, of course, the government does so many things. But I think to own the project so that it is your responsibility, whether or not you're getting funded."[63]

This church leader is quick to identify some of the major challenges resulting from a sustainable Catholic and government multi-disciplinary agenda which places prevention as a key component. Raising awareness of those vulnerable segments of society, here identified as people on ART and AIDS orphans, the Kenyan government is called to provide material support for PLWHA, while the Church is called to provide spiritual support. On the topic of AIDS orphans, the subject reflected:

> But [the government leaders] are trying to provide support at least in terms of orphans. They have now come up with a fund whereby they are trying to—they are piloting it in several areas where any family that is willing to adopt or take in a child, foster child, you will be getting some money per month to support the upkeep of that child, rather than just stick the money in institutions. You know, we have almost close to two million orphans and we can't put up enough institutions—it's too expensive. So they are trying the approach where the children are fostered in homes because of issues in the child adjusting. You know, because even a child growing up in an institution also has its

> own problems. So if those children can grow up in homes, they can reduce the problem afterwards. But the funding of course is not adequate, they give just about 2,000 shillings per month. It's not enough, not at all. But at least it's something.[64]

This self-conscious evaluation of government efforts to address the pressing concern of AIDS orphans clearly demonstrates that the state, supported by religious institutions—chief among them the Catholic Church and church affiliated organizations—assume a form of symbiosis in dealing with prevention throughout Kenya.

Concerning the practical crisis of disease prevention, the twofold question remains as to whether the Catholic Church can rise to meet the needs of the population of Nairobi affected by HIV and AIDS without the aid of the state; and whether the state can serve its vulnerable population without the support of the Catholic Church? After all, there are competing interests in HIV and AIDS prevention such as donor funding, and there is also an overlap of interests from the political, to the ethnic, to the cultural, to the religious. Stated quite succinctly in the words of this Catholic interlocutor, regarding how effective prevention has been from the Catholic perspective, "everything just clashes."[65] The subject continued:

> Initially, there was this urgency. We need more information how to deal with it. I think with the ARV's now, things seem to have kind of settled. We are managing it. But it is a false calm. Because if you are working on the ground, and you go and see the number of orphans, the number of people infected, then you realize nothing really has changed. It's a long-term problem that needs to be supported. You know the focus has moved elsewhere. But we still have people who have to live with it for the rest of their lives. Those orphans are permanent. You can't bring back their parents. They have to be taken care of up until a point where they can be able to stand on their own two feet. So if you're an orphaned and you're one year today, you need another eighteen years for somebody to take care of you until you are able to stand—even eighteen you're not really standing on your own two feet. But at least it's better than nothing. So I think it's a false calm. I really think that attention still needs to go on HIV, so that people are not complacent and just think, "Things are ok. Things are under control, it's no longer happening." But it is.[66]

This church leader's critical assessment of prevention efforts as being historically motivated by religious and social urgency resonates with the AIDS epidemic being presented here as a crisis, particularly with the view that the disease has been addressed and that prevention efforts have been successful. Because of the availability of ARV's, as the subject noted, there is a "false calm," though a silent epidemic remains an epidemic nonetheless. Thus, the crisis of prevention and the ongoing social consequences are all the more real, threatening, and complex from a theological perspective.

Echoing the fear of complacency, one priest identifies a root cause of why prevention efforts have failed to garner and sustain international attention. He noted, specifically for the Church's strategic aims in prevention, "it becomes harder to leverage resources in response to HIV and AIDS. . . . It's harder to get partners and donors to support HIV and AIDS programs because the awareness is quite strong—or the perception is quite strong, that we've basically dealt with the issue. It's no longer a crisis."[67] Here, his concern stems from the fact that prevention programs gave the population of Kenya ample background education on disease transmission from a physiological standpoint.

This provides the population of Nairobi with a false sense of calm, leading to the belief that the epidemic is no longer a crisis that needs advocacy, care, and treatment. A priest mentioned that, "I have a fear, though, for the future in the sense that this diminishing level of commitment interests, which also affects the amount of resources available, I think would have a negative impact if something doesn't change." Spelling out his major concern in prevention, he continued, "I think there is a slackening of commitment probably, as I said earlier on, caused by the fact that there is this erroneous perception that HIV/AIDS is taken care of."[68]

The Catholic Church as simultaneous agent of divine evangelization and agent of human empowerment has a decidedly important role to play in HIV and AIDS prevention, which began in the 1980's and continues even today. In the area of advocacy, the Church as health-care provider and major presence in the arena of politics—both locally in Nairobi and internationally—can positively attend to those living with infection through effective prevention efforts directed toward the AIDS epidemic in Nairobi.

Prevention as *Kairos*

Though the state of prevention in Kenya—especially in the early days of the epidemic—represents a crisis and a common challenge for all religious leaders in Nairobi, there have been some promising trends that might best be considered as *kairos*. Reflecting on the historical presence of the Church in health care throughout Kenya, one Catholic official acknowledged, "the fact that a lot of hospitals are run by Christians, we have a lot of faith-based health-care centers. So a lot of them have taken up distribution of ARV's. When you look at taking care of orphans, people living with HIV—the faith-based response is very good."[69] This history of the Catholic Church providing resources in the form of health care—and for HIV specifically, the distribution of ARV's—is important to acknowledge about prevention since it demonstrates Catholicism as a steward of both body and soul.

As a major figure in the local communities, the Church and its leadership are actively called to provide prevention programs at the grassroots level, meaning that clergy must negotiate with the respective societies to facilitate change. Reflecting on the overlap between the Church and the local community, this Catholic educator states, "They are working together. I think churches work so closely with the communities. There is no competition. The Churches need the community and the community needs the Churches."[70] In this model, the Church is a critical part of the local community and the local community is a critical part of the Church. Neither can realistically exist without the other.

"And a lot of people go to church. Churches are full every Sunday. They work in harmony. I don't see any competition. And actually, even for the pastoral visits, the Church would require the community . . . and the congregation, for the pastoral visits, and all that," the subject continued on the importance of religion in the lives of Kenyans, "Churches and communities are just—you know they are grassroots. They are there where the people are. So you can't ignore them—it's like almost you have to work with a church to get anywhere. It's a good base to work from."[71] That the Church works within the local communities in harmony is heartening, as religious leaders meet the needs of those living with HIV in the patient's own terms and oftentimes in their own homes. The grassroots response to the epidemic through its communal activity in prevention is being bolstered and even conceptually clarified by its association with the Catholic Church.

This view is further supported by another member of church clergy who said, "what I would notice as significant is not been much talked about, is at the grassroots level the response of the religious community is very practical. It's providing care, sustenance."[72] In what might be best described as triage, Catholic Church affiliated grassroots organizations seem to be at the forefront of prevention strategies in Nairobi. This is a notable development, as Catholic figures working in the field are compelled by theological as well as practical impulses. What then follows is less of a focus on magisterial statements regarding church objectives on HIV and AIDS prevention and more of an emphasis on how to really help, aid, and accompany the human person living with HIV infection. The priest continued, "They will do what is needed to save lives or to respond to needs."[73]

The Catholic response to HIV prevention in Kenya can then be seen to include a very practical, lived human dimension that incorporates elements of Catholic social teaching with the understanding that humans make mistakes. And this is where the Catholic Church bridges the conceptual divide between its divine mission and its human nature through its position as health-care provider. "Here in Kenya, a very large percentage of health care is done by religious congregations. A huge percentage," said another Catholic leader working in the field of prevention and grassroots advocacy. "Obviously, HIV is a medical condition so consequently, religious congregations wherever they are throughout the country are not only caring for persons with other diseases, but also persons with HIV."[74]

The fact that the Catholic Church is a major figure in HIV prevention and health-care positions the religious institution in somewhat of a dual manner. This may shed some light on how Catholic strategies in this field represent the appointed time for God's presence, not necessarily in the sense that there is to be some form of divine intervention which will change how people view prevention of HIV and AIDS. Rather, Catholic leaders throughout Nairobi are called to perform God's work in many ways through acts of compassion, justice, mercy, advocacy, hospitality, and outreach.

Just as there are many different elements to the Catholic overarching strategy in dealing with HIV and AIDS in Nairobi, so too are there many different ways of utilizing church leaders in the field of prevention. One Catholic priest and educator sees his writing as a way of making people aware of the disease, which is a critical step in preventing its transmission. "Well, in many ways I would say that personally much of my own engagement in HIV and AIDS has come through writing. So I see that as my own responsibility to write about—for audiences within the Church and outside on issues of HIV and AIDS and how this should shape, affect how we understand ourselves as communities, as Christians," he remarked. "So I see that as a very important role that I play as a religious person is bringing HIV/AIDS into theological perspective and focus. For me that's very important."[75]

The lasting effect of such efforts in the area of prevention serves to educate much of the Catholic population of Nairobi on risk prevention, disease transmission, and access to resources for those infected and affected by the epidemic. The Catholic response to prevention, the subject concluded, "has been significant from the Catholic perspective. The volume of materials that have been generated by Catholic bodies . . . I think is phenomenal, and this I think has been part of the strategy of responding."[76] Prevention, in this form, is an opportunity to raise awareness, not only in Nairobi, but throughout Kenya in general, representing God's decisive action in averting future HIV and AIDS infection.

These religious leaders in Kenya's capital and most populous city aim to meet the people where they live in order to provide care for the body and spirit. This multidimensional, multi-sectorial approach to prevention including grassroots initiatives and advocacy constitutes a holistic endeavor by the Catholic Church, one that looks to the future with hope, as a *kairos*. "My hope for the future, of course is a day when we will not have to live with HIV. When we don't have to deal with it. But in the meantime, we have the information so we need to use it to our benefit," responded the Catholic educator involved in higher education. "We are not like we were 20 years ago, not knowing what had hit us."[77]

"There is hope. I would think for people living with HIV, or even for our society, I can see there is hope. We're not where we were 20 years ago, we are moving forward," one subject declared, considering the prospect for the future. "So we just need to work toward reducing and eradicating HIV—because it's possible. It's one of the preventable diseases, so we shouldn't be getting infected by something we can actually prevent."[78] Prevention remains a field where there has been dramatic improvement over the past twenty years, but an area where there is much more work to be done. In a self-reflexive conclusion, the subject critically assessed the present situation in Kenya looking to the place of aid organizations, saying:

> What I can say, we are appreciating the work that a lot of NGO's and FBO's are doing to highlight different areas that have been neglected or have to be brought out. And with all this work that everybody is doing—the CBO's, FBO'S, NGO's, schools, everybody—I think we are seeing synergy between all these different groups and that's great. And the fact that it's not competition, nobody is trying to outdo each other. There is still so much work that needs to be done there.[79]

Regarding the lasting influence of the Catholic Church and its strategic objectives pertaining to prevention, the official sees the Church as a powerful figure in the field yet humble in its charge to provide care for people living with HIV and AIDS in Nairobi. The subject continued:

> The Churches are still doing a great job, they have always—they have gone to places where even the government doesn't even venture, in very remote areas you'll always find a church. So the importance of the Church should never be underestimated. Of course the Churches don't know how to blow their trumpets. So they continue doing it from a very pastoral [concern]—but the government is beginning to recognize the faith-based sector, especially in health.[80]

That the government is beginning to look to the faith-based and the Catholic-based voice of advocacy and grassroots organization is an interesting development since the government and religious prevention programs overlap in terms of providing a basic standard of health care to those living with infection as well as to those who are negatively affected by the epidemic. The government, in seeking input and insight from Catholic leaders is paving a new and innovative way forward with this multi-sectorial approach in the *kairos* of prevention.

A church leader further describes the relationship of the Catholic Church to the private sector in health care and prevention efforts, observing:

> And that's why the National AIDS Control Council [NACC] now called in the faith-based [sector]. Before they were concentrating on pharmaceuticals, the business sector, the public sector—but now they are realizing that the Church,

> though it is silent, they operate silently. But their contribution is great and sometimes the contribution of the Church is not commercial-based. Because if it's pharmaceuticals, it would be profits. But the Churches are not doing it to get anything in return. So that's a very important areas to tap in on the good will of the Church and really support them where you can. Because a lot of genuine projects—taking care of orphans—sometimes it's done on a voluntary basis. They don't get anything in return, they're not even paid. In fact, they use their own resources. So the faith-based sector needs to be supported and given it its due recognition.[81]

In the subject's estimation of the scene, Nairobi, all Catholics should come to the aid of those grassroots organizations providing both physical and pastoral care to Kenyans affected by HIV. Ever the champion of affirming the inherent dignity of the human person even in the face of intense suffering, Catholic institutions engaged in the field of prevention and health care should be recognized as actively attending to the various practical dimensions of the pandemic—such as dealing with AIDS orphans or the pharmaceutical companies, as the subject noted. In acknowledging the Church as a grassroots activist, a political presence, health-care provider, and religious presence, Catholic leaders in Nairobi in this research identify several of the major challenges that, when reconceptualized, can actually be seen as opportunities to provide care and treatment to Kenyans living through the AIDS epidemic.

To conclude this section, in passing from darkness to light, Catholic leadership living, working, teaching, and ministering in the field of prevention in Nairobi see their position as twofold. On the one hand, they are charged with providing spiritual care to people living with HIV and AIDS. On the other hand, they are called to provide physical care through the *kairos* of prevention. When considering the intersection of the body and the soul, education then presents itself as a somewhat interrelated yet distinct topic for analysis, one to which this chapter now turns.

Education as Crisis

"Probably among the young people I would say they are caught in a Catch-22 situation. You know, these are people who are exposed so much to modern life. And then you are in a society that—you know they are trying to get their foot in the exposure to media, to what is going on around them," reflexively noted one Catholic professor.[82] This account of the experience of young adults in Kenya is striking, in that it addresses several of the important elements that situate the Kenyan Catholic response to HIV and AIDS as a crisis. Not only are there issues of belonging and kinship with an implicit acknowledgment of the tension between the Church, family, and media, but the undercurrent of ethnicity also colors the particular indigenous understanding of the disease and its impact on education.

To set the scope, education as crisis looks to three distinct yet interrelated dimensions of the Catholic response to HIV and AIDS. First, this section reviews the historical significance of Christianity in the field of education—specifically, that church leaders point to a fracturing of Christian teaching, in general, that has led to some confusion regarding the diseases, in general, particularly during the early days of the epidemic. Second, it considers the impact of ethnicity on education, as views pertaining to the various ethnic groups that comprise the Kenyan population influence on how the disease is understood, which, at its very base, is a challenge of education. Third, the section examines the social dilemma of poverty and the difficulty in establishing and supporting education programs.

As a religious institution, the Catholic Church is an important presence in the arena of public and private education in Kenya and so its influence is felt in several different ways. Yet, it is not alone in terms of Christian denominations teaching about HIV and AIDS. This can lead to very confusing and even conflicting opinions concerning how the disease is spread. Remarking on the intrareligious Christian teaching regarding HIV transmission and its influence in the educational sector, one Jesuit priest acknowledged that the Catholic Church is one of the "historical mainline churches . . . missionary founded churches, which are basically extensions of parent bodies. The Catholics, for example, the Methodists, the Anglicans, the Presbyterians—all of these would be mainline churches."[83] These prominent churches, early on, established places of worship, hospitals, and even schools, which became centers of education and evangelization.[84]

However, once Christian teaching was enculturated within the local communities, there arose what are known as African independent churches where a charismatic leader preaches his or her own interpretation of scripture to their congregation with no oversight or magisterium. One Jesuit remarked, "very early on in the history of Christianity in Africa there was also the element of independence where you had independent churches emerging. They were not necessarily connected or haven't broken away from some parent body." He continued:

> But beyond that you've had this situation where there has been a massive growth of religious affiliation of all kinds of categories—Pentecostal, Evangelical, Charismatic—but with little or no connection as a body. So it is a process of continuous fragmentation where churches emerge. So at some point it simply becomes down to the emergence of a leader or someone who considers he or she has something to offer and founds a church, which he or she becomes solely responsible for. Which in a sense can function as some kind of a franchise. You know, you have some of these churches where they have—their branches are planted across the continent and it's a franchise really. There's a pastor who is endorsed to use that brand. You have, like "Winner's Chapel" next door, the "Redeemed Evangelical Mission," "Christ Embassy."

> These are sort of continental and global franchises—brands—that are replicated locally. So, there's really no logic to it, and it's not a process that is regulated. It simply just proliferates depending on personalities, particular circumstances.[85]

This development becomes problematic from an educational standpoint, as these AIC leaders, officials, and clergy began to internalize church teachings and later adapt them for their own ministries. This priest understands that these independent churches can and indeed do tailor their teachings and pastoral care to the needs of the immediate members of the Church. The result is that, on social issues such as education, the AIC's cater to the needs of members in a rather closed circle where welfare and social provisions are made for its constituent members. "It could be assisting children of members with education, it could be counseling for women, but it's limited to their circle of affiliates—which is a different approach from what you might call the more established, historical churches who tend to be more broad in their outlook with regard to how they respond to some of these social issues," said the priest. "So I wouldn't say that these small churches, the newer churches are not socially minded. They are, except they are more focused on their immediate communities."[86] This last remark brings into the discussion the inherent tension between the mainline churches and the independent churches, such that the focus on the needs of the AIC congregations must necessarily be narrower in scope than the larger denominations.

The priests and clergy from the different Christian traditions assume drastically different positions in providing education since the opinions and teachings of the leader become the accepted teaching and mode of education for the church congregation in general. "A lot of people go to church. So their understanding will also be the understanding of the Church," he concluded. "Of course the Catholic Church takes a bit of conservative attitude about HIV, so a lot of people would follow the Church's teachings."[87]

When incorporated into church teaching, what the priest says and teaches about such topics as HIV and AIDS etiology and transmission, when coupled with the priest as moral authority can reinforce negative stereotypes on sexuality and gender, an issue to be taken up in the concluding chapter. Consequently, if the priest or religious official is uninformed about the biomedical dimensions of the disease, the congregation will often remain uninformed as well. This creates a troubling landscape for education regarding HIV and AIDS. In the words of the Jesuit educator, "standing in the position as priests and leaders within their community, they make pronouncements about HIV and AIDS which people take seriously, but which sometimes I fear could be poorly informed, with regards to prevention, or with regards to church policy or teaching positions."[88] Education, therefore, is a very important area of church activity in order to make people aware of how HIV and AIDS is actually transmitted and contracted. As religious leaders, priests are in an influential position to provide this education to their congregations in a faithful and factually correct manner, though the impetus is up to the specific church official to educate themselves about the disease.

Next, culture and ethnicity play an important part in how education can be successful in teaching people in Nairobi about the risk of infection and how to treat the symptoms of the disease. On the topic of kinship and belonging, though confessional Catholics can find common ground in their own religious traditions, there are different ethnic and cultural notions of how the disease is spread. This can thwart Western education models—particularly among the over forty identified ethnic groups throughout Kenya.[89] As one Catholic official on the topic of ethnicity said:

> You know, it really depends a lot on the community. What can I say? I come from a community that surrounds Nairobi. So a lot of their practices are where there was a lot of missionary influence. So if somebody is sick, they go to hospital. Among the Kikuyu community, you are put in the mortuary. They will only come to see you, get you. You know, we have communities where you get the body, and the body sleeps at home. Our community doesn't do that. So you'll pick the body—the day of the burial you'll go to the mortuary. If there is any viewing, it is done at the mortuary. Once that is done, the casket is closed and you go for a Christian burial. And, so there are no rituals.[90]

Even with a confessional self-identification as Christian, some ethnic groups, such as the Kikuyu, treat and understand rituals—as we see here with burials—in a certain light as well as with a certain responsibility that may conflict with more foundational Catholic teachings. This development can make educational initiatives difficult to implement in changing how certain ethnic groups perceive the presence of HIV and AIDS in their own communities. The subject continued:

> Depending on which ethnic background you come from, there is a way you view disease. There are those who will think that you've been cursed, somebody has bewitched you, somebody has looked at you with an evil eye. Then there are those who will think that it is a disease and disease full stop. So go to hospital. Then even among us, we also have religions—the African indigenous religions—there are several sects that do not believe in Western medicine. They believe in—not Western, let's say conventional medicine. They believe in prayer and faith. They'll pray for you until you get healed. So that definitely interferes with treatment and management of HIV. Because if you get sick, you're not taken to hospital. The children are not vaccinated. So again, there are things like polio—and that's dangerous. So the child grows up without any immunity, and the police have been trying to deal with it. If a case like that is heard, they are reported and actually arrested. Mostly what happens is that the children are sick, they are not taking the children to hospital, they are praying for the children. So if you are discovered, it is considered criminal activity. But

> you know that's an issue of faith. But what about that cases where it's not discovered? The child may just die at home for something that could have been treated. Yeah, so then the other issue is the faith healing for people who believe in faith healing. And a lot of—I don't know whether they are taking advantage of the desperation—a lot of churches are coming up and there are those who are genuine. But there are those that, miracles and crusades and all that. And people stop taking their ARV's because they've been prayed for. So it's kind of delicate, faith healing. It confuses people and it can interfere with the management of HIV. Because those who are taking ARV's stop taking it because they have been prayed for and they believe that they are cured. And that will really interfere with your CD-4 count and the process. Because it's a regimen of taking the drugs. So once you stop it becomes a problem.[91]

This apparent disconnect between ethnicity and religion highlights many of the overlapping challenges for education in Nairobi about HIV and AIDS, which supports the assertion that education—especially incomplete or misinformed education—can represent a crisis for people living with infection, as the subject notes. This focus on culture can overshadow church activity from how health care and health-care providers are perceived, to how neonatal care is provided to prevent MTCT, to many other areas that fundamentally deal with education and familiarizing Kenyans with the vocabulary of HIV and AIDS.

With the dimension of culture in dealing with education, this Catholic official names many of the themes already presented—diverse and competing church teaching on the epidemic, and the role of ethnicity in understanding the disease—the subject identifies one other concern in the educational discourse, that of faith healers—self-professed miracle workers who serve to problematize the discourse regarding HIV and AIDS education in Kenya. While certain ethnic groups do consult local faith healers (KiSwahili, *mganga* or *daktari wa kienyeji*), the presence of faith healers who are often tied to their very own AIC presents a major challenge for Catholic educators in disseminating factually and scientifically sound information about the AIDS epidemic.

Due to the tense relationship between some religious leaders and education—not just Catholics, but also independent church leaders who claim to heal their congregations of disease—the heart of the crisis becomes conflicting accounts of disease origin and transmission which can lead to confusion among persons religious regarding the epidemic. On the effects of popular ethnic opinion among the Catholic population of Nairobi, one church leader remarked regarding education initiatives, is that they "can go very negative or very positive. So it really depends on the opinion of the pastor and that's not a very good thing sometimes."[92]

One final area of consideration vis-à-vis the crisis of education in Catholicism looks to the place of poverty as a significant challenge for teaching about the disease. This, of course, treats education from a religious standpoint as well as from a human, practical standpoint. "I would say poverty is a big issue. Poverty remains a big issue, when people have little option—than to engage in transactional sex. It's an issue," a Jesuit priest noted, as he described some of the major obstacles to Catholic education in Kenya. "It is also compounded by this negative, or rather erroneous impression that it's not a threat anymore. The myths have not gone away about HIV and AIDS—how you contract it, how you cure it, sleeping with underage girls. So I would put it down to that factor, of lack of socioeconomic resources."[93]

Not only does poverty inhibit educational efforts by reducing material resources but it also influences the conditions under which risk-behavior flourishes—namely transactional sex. Sex workers represent one of the largest demographics of new infection.[94] Poverty in Nairobi is therefore a significant issue for those at risk of becoming infected since, as the priest noted above, myths and incorrect information surround popular opinions on how HIV is contracted, treated, and—even according to one widespread belief—cured. Education in terms of prevention, then, may be hampered by such prevailing opinion especially when compounded by the influence of independent churches and ethno-cultural understandings of HIV and AIDS. Taken as a whole, all three dimensions of the crisis overlap in some very problematic ways. As another church leader asserted:

> Yes, of course, poverty is a problem. Because poverty is at the basis of quite a bit of the transmission. If I am living in these informal communities, surrounding cities—Nairobi, for example,—and I'm in rented accommodation, and getting food is difficult. Obviously, women would feel that, "Well, there's something that I don't need money for to do." And that is prostitution. So I can go into commercial sex. Because I don't need any let papers or qualifications or anything. I don't need any money, resource—I just need my own body. So poverty is often—how to put it? People who are living below the poverty line often have no way of getting money except by, I'm talking about women now, except through commercial sex. Now, obviously that's the possibility for the transmission of the virus.[95]

While this excerpt addresses many of the social dimensions of disease transmission—such as gender roles and sexuality, which will be treated in chapter 4—it paints a tragic picture of how poverty has impeded education efforts in Nairobi, leading people to engage in risk behavior despite education by the Catholic Church. This goes back to a moralistic reading of how one is infected with HIV and AIDS. The sheer desperation of people living in poverty in Nairobi is staggering. "Poverty compounds everything, every situation in life," the subject concluded.[96]

One final note on the crisis of education in Kenya's capital. Where the three areas examined in this section—churches, ethnicity, and poverty—

cover a wide range of ancillary topics, they are themselves not mutually exclusive. As one Catholic educator engaged in inter-faith dialogue observed as one of the largest hurdles for effective education, "Looking at Kenya, I would say partially it could be poverty in some areas. That vicious cycle of poverty, where people don't see an outlet to it."[97] Again the issue of poverty and desperation plays a large part in addressing the challenge that church leaders have in providing essential teaching programs and educational policies. In addition to poverty in general, this Catholic leader makes the conceptual leap to the intersection of poverty and ethnicity. "Some pastoralist communities practice polygamy. You know, if you're married as a fourth, fifth, or seventh wife—you don't have much rights. The man is the very dominant figure and you don't question anything he does," the subject continued. "There are certain, there are quite a number of factors that are causing [HIV and AIDS] to spread. But, of course for the middle class and others there are different reasons. Not poverty, but among the poorer areas, you'll find it will be a lot of what I mentioned before of the vicious cycle of poverty, cultural practices."[98]

Thus, the Catholic Church faces many practical challenges regarding HIV and AIDS education, chief among them the institutional history of Christianity, ethnicity, culture, and poverty. Yet, while these systematic challenges represent a crisis for the Church in Nairobi, Catholic leaders can act as agents of change so that, in the strategic objectives of education, they move past the practical difficulties of the present crisis to illuminate church teaching and policy.

Education as *Kairos*

Having examined the challenges facing church representatives on HIV and AIDS education in Nairobi in the previous section, we now look to Catholic social teaching as a potentially transforming presence in how Kenyan Catholics understand the current epidemic and people living with infection. Stated quite succinctly by one subject, "I mean, there are controversies about the morality in the material, education has been an area of huge contribution from the Church."[99] This education, however, does not only exist and operate in classrooms, conferences, and workshops, which aim to familiarize the general population of Nairobi about how the disease is actually transmitted. Rather, these efforts involve changing the way people view and treat people who are HIV positive irrespective of whether they are Catholic or not. Said one nun working in health care on the topic of educational initiatives affiliated with the Catholic Church, "I believe these to be justice issues. These are very much part of the Church's role in communicating to Catholics how to live the Christian way of life. The compassion. The compassion for people."[100]

This transition from education as instruction to education effectively based in justice and compassion for individuals living with illness is a very fascinating theological development. It involves educating the person as a whole, both practically and religiously. It also calls all Catholics to live their faith.[101] Such a strategy for the Catholic Church and for church officials involves addressing and meeting the fundamental problems facing those educators who deal with HIV and AIDS in their own lives or in their communities.

One major factor of this education as opportunity—as *kairos*—requires the Church to exercise its position as a social institution, especially in the realm of politics most readily accomplished through advocacy. The Catholic Church as a community of individuals living in the social environment of Nairobi has the distinct power to influence how people perceive their fellow Kenyans living with HIV and AIDS. In one stunning turn of events, an orphanage in Nairobi successfully pursued litigation against the Kenyan government for discriminating against students infected with HIV. Asserted the church leader involved in the litigation process, "when President [Mwai] Kibaki was elected as president, his first campaign priority was free education for children in primary schools." Yet this campaign promise did not account for how people living with infection are popularly viewed by the rest of society. "Throughout 2003 the first year of his time as president, no matter how many times our social workers went to the government schools near [the orphanage], strangely the classes were always full."[102] With full classes, students from the orphanage with HIV could not legally attend classes. "We got the message—discrimination against these children who were living with HIV," the official continued. "So the children took the government of Kenya to court and won the case. So we pushed for education without discrimination."[103]

This legal precedent singles out the dimension of discrimination in the public's view toward people living with HIV and AIDS and helps to clarify the Catholic Church's position as policy-maker and agent of change and empowerment in Kenya. Particularly in the field of education, the Church and members of clergy have considerable influence to bring about the *kairos* of God's appointed presence through their advocacy and political presence, both individually and collectively.

In the estimation of another Catholic working with church-based education initiatives, education is an effective remedy in affirming the inherent dignity of people negatively affected by the epidemic since it also leads to examining broader structural issues—such as prevention, poverty, popular culture, and ingrained ethno-cultural perceptions of the disease. "Now, an education—knowledge is power. So we need to use that information that we have to try and eradicate [HIV and AIDS], or prevent, or manage it," stated a Catholic involved in higher education. "It's unfortunate, a lots of things interfere—like what we would say about cultural, traditional beliefs, socioeconomics—there are a lot of environmental issues. But at least, once we have the knowledge, we need to just use what we have at our disposal to look for a solution that can work for the majority of the people."[104]

For this leader, the Catholic Church is in a prominent position to address many of the major issues facing disease prevention through education. As a social and a religious establishment, the Church is distinctively suited to combat inaccurate views about HIV and regarding people living with the virus. As educator, the Catholic Church can actively set the tone and scope of the national discourse surrounding the epidemic, accompanying those affected by HIV and AIDS, and seeking the preferential option for those living on the margins of society.

Looking to the ethic of compassion based in the acknowledgment of human suffering, this leader indicates the root causes of why the disease continues to spread even in light of large scale education and prevention programs. Yet, there is a surprising tone of hope in the *kairos* of God's activity, that the Church will work diligently to empower those living with the disease in its position as policy-maker and proponent of advocacy through education. Catholics are thus called to not only engage in advocacy and perform grassroots outreach to people infected, but the Catholic community of faithful serves as an important reminder for millions of Kenyans living in and around Nairobi as well as in other rural areas throughout Kenya, that they have a voice and can demand change.

Because of its consistent presence, the Church historically serves as a mediator between the Church and the state in the form of education. On the topic of outreach, one subject noted that a significant area of Catholic Church activity is in the form of "outreach toward the less privileged, those who need. So it's a good base for mobilizing communities to respond."[105] The Church as social actor and agent of empowerment for those living with HIV and AIDS lends its influence to Church as educator, particularly as it has tremendous influence in the lives of the contextual and living community of believers. "Inasmuch as whatever opinion it has of HIV, it still is the same Church that reaches out to the poor, to those who are in need of help and encourages the community surrounding it to do so and the people who go to church," the Catholic official critically reflects. "So I think it's—it's, most of the mainstream churches are doing well in that area."[106]

This assessment of church identity and presence in the local community bears further consideration, since it illuminates the extensive scope of Catholic-affiliated activity—not only in education, both overlapping in a interdisciplinary way in the fields of advocacy and community mobilization. Active in many local communities, the Catholic Church and church leaders, officials, and clergy specifically, are duly charged with faithfully serving their congregations in any number of ways, motivated by an emphasis on education as a productive channel for change as *kairos* moment through individual and collective action. Stated differently, church leaders seek to create an environment that fosters the dignity of those individuals living with disease thereby bringing about the appointed time for God's decisive action through their own work in the field of education.

In this way, they are living agents of God's divine presence throughout Nairobi. And while there are those priests and members of clergy that are fomenting negative, moralistic views about those living with the virus, it would seem that the overwhelming majority of Kenyan Catholic leadership interviewed for this project strive to disabuse their fellow Catholics in the use of these pejorative judgments. When formulated positively, education effort—presented here as one dimension of *Kairos*—can and indeed are changing how people perceive HIV and AIDS as well as those individuals living with infection.

Where the Catholic Church actively pursues its goals in the area of policy and advocacy for both religious and secular education, there remains the theological mandate to provide effective education to the society within which the Church operates. After all, Proverbs 9:9 states, "Give instruction to the wise, and they will become wiser still; teach the righteous and they will gain in learning."[107] One of the complex issues related to HIV and AIDS education from a religious perspective involves viewing the place of sexuality in negative terms. While this topic will be taken up in significant detail in the concluding chapter, it is worth addressing here briefly that church teaching, sexuality, and education are intimately related. The Catholic nun examines this issue when she self-consciously acknowledged, "the Catholic Church here has had a stand against having components of education dealing with HIV and sexuality in the public curriculum. And it still, as far as I know, is not very clear."[108] Even though the Church is aware that there are issues stemming from issues of sexuality, and with the majority of church clergy and leadership being overwhelmingly male, church doctrine on sexuality seems to be systematically problematic. As we shall see, this is not an issue specific to Catholicism in Kenya but one that the Muslim population also acknowledges.

"That is the big reason why the teaching of the Catholic Church is skewed a bit, and also why religious education is skewed," she affirmed, noting that there is an imbalance in church teaching regarding sexuality. "And so therefore, the whole issue of including sexuality and HIV in the curriculum has been contested very much by the Catholic Church."[109] Since church leaders are responsible for curriculum development, this stinging critique on the basis of excluding teaching about sexuality seems a negative trend, one which might be better placed as a challenge or crisis for the Church in the time of AIDS for the Catholics of Nairobi. However, the very fact that a female Catholic leader is willing to openly find fault with religious education as being partially "skewed" against teaching on sexuality in the HIV and AIDS curriculum is heartening.

As a matter of critical self-analysis, the Church is called to exert its influence to all sectors of the Kenyan society, and issues of sexuality in education are disturbingly important in the discourse surrounding the epidemic in Nairobi. This is in part true because talking about infection means talking about sex—not simply transmission due to sexual intercourse, but also the ingrained gender roles and their imbalance that allow for women to be considered as less than men.

Again, addressing the balance of education and church teaching, Catholic teaching, and sexuality, the female church representative looks to the model of Jesus Christ as providing the necessary clarification between the three seemingly contentious dimension regarding church doctrine. In considering the person of Jesus Christ, education—and even education dealing with the problematic issues of sexuality from a religious perspective—can indeed be seen as a *kairos* for God's activity. The subject challenges the Church to be the operative agent of God's decisive action on earth, saying "I would hope that the pastoral aspect of Jesus' message would now have the prominence, and that sexuality would come into a much more balanced context in the Church's teaching. That's what my hope would be."[110] Maintaining the balance between two extremes, this religious official calls the Church to structure its education objectives with sexuality in mind. Reflecting on the official church policy pertaining to HIV and sexuality, the subject next asserted, "I'd hope that the balance between teaching and practice would also be more pastoral—because the doctrine was the last word."[111]

This observation echoes the divide between doctrinal teaching and practical responses to HIV and AIDS in Kenya, which at times can be drastically different and legitimated by different proximate causes, depending on the source of the teaching. However, overshadowing this entire discussion is the influence of Jesus Christ and his teachings.

In conjuring an image of this compassionate Jesus, the Catholic Church is reminded that the Church is not only a political figure. It is also not only a religious institution with its foundation in divine scripture and tradition. Rather, the Church is a collective of individuals who have very basic human needs. With the example of Jesus who educated humanity through his compassion, this vision of Christ relates, interacts, and radically changes the lives of those whom he encounters. So too, the Catholic Church as an agent of *kairos* has the ability to empower and forever change the lives of those individuals living with HIV and AIDS in Nairobi.

This conception of Jesus as a compassionate educator calling people to live their true humanity maintains a creative tension between church teaching, sexuality, and the actual implementation of education from a religious viewpoint. Yet, in the eyes of Catholic leaders actually living in Nairobi and facing daily the long-term effect of practical, lived responses to HIV and AIDS by the Church, compassion by clergy and religious officials can act as a way of bringing about the *kairos* that AIDS education needs primarily through personal interaction with people infected with HIV. In this way, Catholic leaders are working to realize God's activity in Nairobi through striking a balance between official church teaching and the lived educational efforts of those individuals working at the grassroots level.

The hope remains for the future that, through individual and combined activity on the part of the Church in Nairobi, Catholics will pave the way for the *kairos* in religious and practical education. However, one of the largest challenges for education remains eliminating the social and physical stigma directed toward those people infected with the disease. For this reason, the next section examines efforts of Catholic leaders in destigmatization and combatting negative public opinion regarding HIV and AIDS in Nairobi.

Destigmatization as Crisis

"It's extremely difficult, if I have HIV and not only am I dealing with the medical challenge but I am looked at by many Catholics as somebody who has acted immorally," the subject continued. "It even goes down to my identity. That I'm condemned. So that is huge."[112] Indeed, stigma is one of the most troubling dimensions of the AIDS epidemic in Kenya. Programs directed toward destigmatization must change popularly held beliefs about the disease, its mode of transmission, and its origin. Topics such as "immorality" and "condemnation" in the above excerpt are all too often negatively attributed to persons infected and this moralistic reading of the virus can even be directed to the family.

Inasmuch as it deals with the opinions that people have about HIV and AIDS and those who have contracted the infection, stigma "remains the most ineluctable, indefinable, intractable problem in the epidemic. Stigma is perhaps the greatest dread of those who live with AIDS and HIV—greater to many even more than the fear of a disfiguring, agonizing and much protracted death."[113] A powerful social force, stigma entails a perception used to create an other-izing binary, one that proposes the categories of "us" and "them." In Nairobi, "them" represents those living with HIV infection. The stigmatizing principle seeks to make sense of how the disease is transmitted and contracted, obscured by the belief in disordered sexuality, taboo, and broken social norms. "Besides the general problem, stigma is still a big problem with regards to HIV and AIDS which then determines people's responses and how they relate to it," said the subject.[114]

Since stigmatization is a social phenomenon—one created, exercised, and reinforced by the people that actually make up the community—stigma itself remains one deeply conflicted element of the AIDS crisis in Kenya. Simply stated, stigma "can be seen as an attribute that discredits the individual, denying full social acceptance, where notions of inclusion and exclusion are firmly brought to the fore."[115] Drawing into focus the other-izing binary of "us" and "them," employing terminologies of exclusion and inclusion in human societies such as Nairobi acts to create divisions within the community, as religiously-reinforced moralistic readings into disease origin and transmission strengthen prevailing notions about modes of infection.

Indeed, it is through stigma that society attaches "a negative social label of disgrace, shame, and prejudice or rejection to a person who differs from us in some way that we experience as running counter to our deeply imbedded values and prejudices."[116] When applied to the AIDS crisis, the result diminishes the humanity of people who live with the virus. This Catholic member of clergy in Kenya's capital city stated further, "there is what I would call disproportionate disapproval, I don't want to use condemnatory [terms], but the element of condemnation is there. And there's this disproportionate disapproval of persons with HIV."[117]

The term this Catholic leader uses to address the effect of stigma toward those living with infection, "disproportionate disapproval," is useful in characterizing the religious response to the epidemic by the Church. As has been explored elsewhere, the Catholic Church has historically been a major figure throughout Kenya—not only in politics, activism, and advocacy—but also in the field of secular and religious education. Church efforts in this field allow religious leaders to disseminate both official and personal views about the disease that, as has been seen, is not always positive. Even though church representatives are held to magisterial teachings which seek to affirm the inherent dignity of all persons everywhere—particularly those living with illness and disease—these teachings can be informed by a particular pastor's personal views and opinions about HIV and AIDS.

For example, homosexuality and homosexual relations carry with them a particular moralistic judgment from the Catholic Church and the church *Catechism*.[118] However, a major theological and pastoral question considers how Catholic leaders can attend to this marginalized section of the Kenyan population who already face legal, social, and religious judgment, sanctions, and stigma.[119] The Catholic representative observed, "homosexuality is a big issue here in Africa, similar to how it was before the 1960s that the facts about homosexuality were just not known."[120] In drawing a parallel between homosexuality in the 1960s in America and in the 1990s in Kenya, this interviewee claims that once HIV and AIDS was associated with homosexuality, it was difficult to shift popular opinion that those who had contracted the disease were necessarily homosexuals.

"But once [the connection between HIV and homosexuality] became known, then still that did not destigmatize homosexuality," the subject continued. This stark evaluation of the apparent disconnect between church teaching and homosexuality does little to ease the stigma that Kenyan society directs in correlating homosexuality and HIV infection. Regarding the effect of this negative perception of homosexuality based in church teaching and culture, the respondent continued, "here it's skewed by the tradition, as it was skewed by tradition in the developed world before the 1960s. So consequently, that's another area of sexuality that is very contentious."[121]

The term "contentious" employed by the subject aptly characterizes some of the major obstacles facing destigmatization efforts on the topic of homosexuality since there are negative cultural, ethnic, social, legal, and not least of all, religious connotations. Stigma, then, reinforces certain patterns of behavior that are socially acceptable, forcing those who do not fully meet the standards set by popular opinion to the fringes of society often surrounded by the shroud of silence and denial. Stigma and silence are intimately related, as humans from all sectors of Kenyan society are expected to live up to some preconceived notion of what it means to behave rightly, even though humans as humans consistently falter in what is expected of them, both socially and religiously.

Then the question arises as to what to make of priests who have contacted HIV and AIDS as religious leaders of the community? How does society perceive these individuals? In the view of one Catholic leader, "in a lot of churches, I think if a clergy person turned out to be HIV positive, the way they would be received would be different . . . a priest is a human being. And they can get infected."[122] This is a striking statement as it depicts Catholic priests as human beings and not above being infected with HIV and AIDS.

Indeed, stigma remains a problem for the church hierarchy, even more so since these infected individuals represent the official Church. Yet there is no reason to believe that religious leaders cannot contract the disease as easily as anyone else. The subject continued, saying that infection among the Catholic leadership is "a new area where other churches would not readily want to talk about clergy being HIV positive. The issues of gay priests—homosexuals—you know there are certain areas that are a bit thorny. So it's kind of treading in a new area, but a very necessary area. Because anybody can get HIV, so where would they go?"[123] This excerpt demonstrates the explicit link between stigma and silence, further strengthening the poignant question of where a HIV positive priest would go for VCT or disclose their status.

Thus, priests as humans are susceptible to disease and are at-risk, though this does little to combat the stigma of popular opinion regarding sexuality. On the social and religious expectation instilled by stigma, on matters such as extra-marital affairs, the subject continued, "it shouldn't happen. And if it does happen, then you have one big explanation to give. Sometimes the Church tends to look at HIV from a moral perspective. It's very hard not to, from a church perspective."[124] Stigma, therefore, acts as a behavior moderator, since faithfully married couples in the Catholic Church in Nairobi should be faithful and should not engage in sexual relations outside of marriage. And yet, extra-marital affairs do occur in both secular and religious contexts, which make stigma—or the perception of a particular standard of living toward which people are meant to live—all the more a significant factor in the crisis of HIV and AIDS.

In terms of stigma directed toward different types of sin, this Catholic interlocutor posed the compelling parallel that, "you'd rather steal—get a bit of funds from the Church—but not a sexual sin. It's easier to shut your eyes on one but not the other. I think one carries more moral judgment."[125] To say that sexual sin carries a different moral weight is intriguing, since such an understanding goes back to the skewed teachings regarding sexuality in the practical implementation of church doctrine addressed earlier. There are many factors that influence the public perception of HIV and AIDS in Kenya including some that are social and others that are religious. In order for the Church to shift the discussion about the epidemic from one that focuses on sexuality to one that calls the Church and its representatives to accompany and attend to all those negatively affected by disease, many of whom contracted the disease through various means.

One other population susceptible to the negative impact of stigma are the families of those infected. Even after the death of those who have succumbed to opportunistic infection, during the burial ceremony there is often silence associated with their legacies. As one Catholic respondent noted, "when it comes to the actual burials, you hardly ever hear the priest mention HIV. There is still silence around if that was the actual cause of death, it's not mentioned."[126] Stigma and silence remain powerful challenges to radically changing how the general public of Kenya perceives the disease. This includes Catholic leaders who are in a distinct position of influence and authority influencing how the constituent Catholic bodies view and approach the disease. The subject sees one benefit for remaining silent at the burials of those who have died from opportunistic infections as the result of AIDS saying, "I think in one way it protects the living. Already they are going through the trauma of losing a loved one. Because the stigma is still there, you don't also want to stigmatize the family further."[127]

As a negative, though intangible dimension of the epidemic in Nairobi, stigma engenders silence to protect the reputation of the family of those who have succumbed to AIDS. "Though, of course it beats the logic—you know that people say that if it is out in the open, people often just say, if somebody died of HIV, just say it," the subject continued. "But you can't say it because of the stigma levels, the environment it still not safe or conducive enough . . . so, few people say it, but not many. Not many. Most of them prefer to just keep it silent."[128] According to this Catholic leader, by consciously not speaking about the illness, the family and church representatives are actually doing a disservice by reinforcing negative views regarding AIDS infection.

These last few lines of the interview demonstrate the lack of transparency in Nairobi, that the current environment is not supportive for talking to people about how one dies from the infection and their legacies. What then occurs and has been occurring throughout sub-Saharan Africa as in other parts of the world throughout the past three decades, is a "conspiracy of silence" to use Donald E. Messer's phrase, a conspiracy that can detract from the memories of those who have died due to complications and opportunistic infection arising from their infection. While burial services might not be the best or most tactful platform for breaking the silence enshrouding the epidemic in Nairobi, the interlocutor clearly noted that, "the priest will just say, 'he died of sickness.' Because even in funerals, you don't say 'Well, he died of cancer' or 'He died of illness.' You know, you don't keep specifying that this was. . . . So people ask, 'Why should then you specify for HIV if you don't specify for the others?' So, sometimes there are all those kind of issues."[129]

Priests and clergy must be educated in the vocabulary of HIV and AIDS so they can thoughtfully and knowledgably speak to their congregations about the stigma associated with the virus as well as how the negative impact that this other-izing behavior can have on people living with infection as well as on their families. Religious leaders assume an influential position to enlighten the Catholic population by again reframing established church teaching into a practical, pastoral, grassroots response to HIV and AIDS in the local communities. The Catholic Church can realize its mission by teaching and witnessing that stigma can yield to understanding, that despair can yield to hope, darkness can yield to light, and above all that this crisis can yield to and be transformed into *kairos*.

Destigmatization as *Kairos*

"Everybody who is working with persons who are living with HIV is aware of the stigma. So insofar as the Catholic Church is working with persons with HIV, they would be aware of the injustice of the stigma," asserted a Catholic nun. "Whenever I get the chance to talk—and I do talk quite a bit—I talk about the injustice of stigma and discrimination."[130] Even though stigma necessarily entails negative dimensions—of discrimination, of injustice as the nun points out—the converse would constitute a *kairos* for the Catholic Church through stigma mitigation as an opportunity to assuage the physical and physiological pain and suffering of those who live with HIV and AIDS infection. This can be accomplished most readily and effectively by church leaders in two major ways, the first theologically and the second practically in terms of how the disease is popularly understood as a medical condition. In actively establishing and pursuing destigmatization initiatives, clergy and church officials can promote the preferential option for those living at the margins of society, notably for this project Kenyans living with HIV and AIDS.

In theological terms, Catholic leaders are charged with the challenge of affirming the inherent dignity of those infected by such a physically debilitating and socially stigmatizing disease. A Jesuit who works in advocacy and education in Nairobi uses scripture to inform his daily work of destigmatization in the local Catholic community with a verse from the Gospel of John 10:10, "I came that all may have life, and have it abundantly."[131] He acknowledged, "that's been the motivating scripture verse. . . . The idea of promoting life in a culture that has been so decimated by death through this disease."[132] Framing the conversation on destigmatization in positive terms—of promoting life in the face of death—is a powerful theological image that truly illuminates the basic dichotomy of the AIDS epidemic in Kenya as a movement from crisis to *kairos*.

Emphasizing the interrelatedness of the Catholic common good tradition, he further stated, "I would say for people who are living with HIV and AIDS, I think there is no doubt any more that we are all part of God's own creation."[133] As a community of believers, Catholics in Nairobi and throughout Kenya are expected to accompany each other in the fullness of Christ, which also entails recognizing the inherent dignity of all humans as created in the image of God or the *imago dei*. Consequently, where stigma is influenced by a popular perception, culturally and socially, Catholics are theologically called to break the chains of stigma. "And the fact that one is infected with or affected by HIV and AIDS, it does not in any way remove a person's dignity," he continued. "And each person is entitled to be treated with respect, with care, and dignity—irrespective of the serostatus of the person."[134] Human dignity must not be diminished by a moral judgment of a person. To judge someone morally would completely contradict the theological mandate of the Catholic Church, or for St. John in the Gospel it would prevent a certain segment of the society from having life "in full."

Reflecting again on the importance of *kairos* as a transformative event, the priest recognized, "I think we've come a long way and I believe that people living with HIV and AIDS are fully integrated into religious communities."[135] This is both a theological as well as a social development. In the early 1980s through the 1990s those who had contracted the disease were met with stigma, silence, discrimination, and isolation. The subject remarked that this has largely changed though it has not been entirely eradicated. "This is not to say that there are not pockets of stigmatization," he confirmed, "but I think there is a greater opening toward the fact that living with HIV and AIDS doesn't in any way diminish a person's integrity nor in any way diminishes her claim on the moral responsibility of the community to offer care and support."[136]

The last point, that seropositive status does not lessen a person's dignity or integrity—nor the responsibility of the society to offer support to all of its members—is fascinating since it proposes a twofold relationship between the individual and the community, based in the common good tradition of Catholicism.[137] Returning to the negative trend of morally judging or condemning people who have contracted HIV and AIDS infection, the Catholic Church has made strides in destigmatization by emphasizing that it is incumbent on individuals to pursue the common good of the community, which then flows back onto its constituent members.[138] When formulated this way, the community is responsible for all of its members, including most notably those affected by disease. It then becomes a matter of social justice for the community to provide care and support to people living with HIV and AIDS in Nairobi. Or, in the words of one representative involved in destigmatization efforts by a Catholic-based NGO in Nairobi, "justice is justice, and any discrimination of any nature is unjust. Whether it's based on race, religion, political affiliation—or in this case, a medical condition."[139]

In establishing the tone of the discourse, the Church is responsible for providing effective teaching, palliative health care, and programs aimed at stigma mitigation for anyone affected by the disease. The community and the individual are, therefore, in a state of symbiosis where the health and social status of the individual is intrinsically tied to the health of the community. From a medical standpoint, one subject noted, "HIV is a medical condition. It's no different from diabetes—or cancer. It's a chronic medical condition and no longer fatal. So consequently, discrimination on that basis is very unjust."[140] To reiterate a point made earlier, there are spiritual and physical dimensions to the HIV and AIDS epidemic in Kenya. Even when examining the medical aspects of the disease—as a chronic condition, treatable but with no known cure—the issue of discrimination based on negative stigma brings into the conversation a distinctly theological notion of what is just and what is unjust.

To discriminate on the basis of seropositive status yet not discriminate against someone who has diabetes or cancer is a very intriguing social phenomenon, one which considers the disease itself and its means of transmission in a decidedly moralistic light. Thus, when viewed as *kairos*, church activity in the realm of destigmatization engages both the physical/medical dimension of the disease as well as its spiritual/theological dimension. Physically, as health-care provider, the Church provides treatment for HIV and AIDS as a medical condition. Spiritually, the Church works to mitigate the discrimination directed toward those living with the disease, through enunciating key objectives aimed at destigmatization. The crossroads of compassion and justice is thus a compelling way to view the *kairos* of stigma reduction.

Compassion here does not mean, the respondent claimed, "differentiating [PLWHA] from others with other medical conditions. But you see, the problem is that it's stigmatized as a medical condition. And it's only a medical condition."[141] In the preceding account, equanimity is proposed for treating people inflicted with any form of disease, as health care in its basic formulation is blind to the social factors and circumstances of the sick. And yet, when it comes to HIV and AIDS, there is a moralistic judgment concerning how the disease was originally contracted. "A major reason for the universality and depth of AIDS-related stigma is undoubtedly the way in which society sees adult HIV infections as resulting from disapproved of behavior and interpreting this in moral terms," writes Fr. Michael Kelly, SJ, in his notable work, *HIV and AIDS: A Social Justice Perspective*.[142] In this moralistic formulation, those acts of social disapproval according to set standards of behavior deserve social punishment in the form of stigma.

As one subject mentioned, from a biomedical perspective, people living with HIV and AIDS, "have a virus, for which at the moment there is no cure. There is only medicine to contain it. That is all."[143] The far-reaching impact of stigma seeks to dehumanize those infected with the virus, which requires compassion from Catholic leaders working in care and treatment to attend to the person with HIV, who are the susceptible to illness and popular opinion. "If I tell you I have diabetes, you'd have compassion for me," the subject continued. But if that same person were to disclose their seropositive status, many people—among them Catholics—might not respond to them compassionately. Concluding, this subject added "It's a moralistic reading into my condition."[144] When concerning HIV and AIDS in Nairobi, morality and medicine maintain a tense relationship. Combatting this stigma and moralistic condemnation is a necessary aim for those Catholics working in the area of health care in order to treat the human person.

By moving beyond HIV and AIDS as a moral issue to an understanding of the disease as a medical condition opens the door for a constructive conversation, one which moves away from discrimination to one which aims to treat the person with dignity. Regarding compassion and equality, the subject continued concerning the state of being seropositive, "There isn't any basis to see me as less equal than you, less in any way regarding services. Whether they're medical services, whether they're employment services. Whether they're religious relationships, whatever. That I'm no different, that I have a medical condition and that's all."[145] Equality of services and of people therefore represents the overarching mandate for Catholic leaders working in both pastoral and medical care.

For instance, regarding children infected with the disease, this Catholic official who oversees an AIDS orphanage in Nairobi remarked, "I don't think about the fact that our children have HIV—it just doesn't enter my mind. They're young people, they're orphans sadly. Their parents have passed away." The subject then said, "We try to give them as close a family life as possible, as they grow up here. We get great joy seeing them grow up and fulfill their potential. It just doesn't enter into any of my relationships, nor my relationships with anybody else with HIV."[146] Representative of the influence and impact of the Catholic Church in Nairobi, the religious response is incumbent on an openness toward those infected with HIV and AIDS—openness to see them as humans, made in the image of God and following in the footsteps of Jesus Christ.

Catholics who move past a moralizing attitude about someone's medical condition help to realize the *kairos* in their lives and the lives of those with HIV, since, according to this subject, Catholics should come to the aid of those infected with "care and treatment. That's compassion. The care and treatment that is done within compassionate context—there is no discrimination, no stigmatization."[147] Since humans are imperfect, Catholic leaders are called to engage the epidemic with a theology of compassion and forgiveness, acknowledging realistic human behavior even through the stigmatization and discrimination toward people infected. Catholic leaders are then called, the subject continued, "because there is stigmatization and discrimination, to get into the justice issue and speak and try to destigmatize the approach to persons with HIV on the basis of justice. There's compassion, but it has to be based on justice."[148]

By stressing the relationship between compassion, destigmatization, and justice, "it is important to remember that although it is possible to initiate action against overt manifestations of discrimination, no public measures or legislation can reach into the human heart, into those depths where prejudice and stigma originate," Fr. Kelly writes. "And this is above all where work to bring about change must be initiated and brought to fulfillment."[149]

As Fr. Kelly rightfully acknowledges, this process has not been an easy one and there are still obstacles to be overcome. Changing popular opinion includes efforts by the Catholic Church in combatting negative views of HIV and AIDS, which at its foundation includes educational initiatives at destigmatization, both intra- and interreligiously. It is also where there is much conceptual overlap between prevention, education, and destigmatization in the holistic approach by Catholics in Nairobi toward those persons negatively affected by the disease. In a marked shift away from denial and silence, some churches are proactively initiating open forums in which matters of HIV and AIDS are forthrightly discussed, often bringing leaders and laity from other Christian denominations together to talk about programs that are working, projects that are failing, and other strategies that might work.

One Catholic representative interviewed for this project spoke in notably positive terms about the openness in discussing the pandemic in the Church, citing, "In our church, they get speakers once in a while to come and talk about HIV. And after we have the speakers talk—they have the mobile clinics for testing [VCT]. The Presbyterian Church has invited me to be a speaker in their church."[150] We have here both theological engagement as well as a practical, pastoral engagement whereby Catholic preachers speak about issues of HIV and AIDS from the pulpit—in the churches of other Christian denominations—and then offer VCT services that meet the needs of both the body and the soul. The subject further stated:

> So during the summer, they have HIV week—I mean, AIDS awareness week. So actually it's a month, every week they bring a preacher who speaks on HIV issues. And that is done in the Church. After they read the bible, the sermon is just on HIV awareness. So I went to the Presbyterian Church and I talked about issues of HIV, creating awareness. So the Church, it's all done very frequently but at least they do—and I know that the Anglican Church, All Saint's Cathedral in Nairobi, they have a needs awareness month when every Sunday they have—there's a theme. So a few churches have become proactive and they have different themes, I know St. Andrew's Presbyterian Church has a theme on disability. So for one whole week, they will have even people with disabilities coming in, creating awareness, talking to the people in the Churches. And I think it's working, because people become aware about issues they would not really concern themselves with.[151]

This intra-religious exchange of ideas and themes points to a key component of the Catholic response to HIV and AIDS in Nairobi. There are complex and interrelated factors at work that church clergy must address so that those negatively affected by the AIDS epidemic may have their dignity and integrity affirmed in the face of sickness and suffering. The Catholic Church is particularly well-suited to address and respond to the myriad concerns of its congregation, by delivering sermons which aim to familiarize its people with the theological and biomedical terminologies of HIV and AIDS, and even provide mobile testing so people can know their status, standing in solidarity against denial, silence, and stigma.

CONCLUSION

In theological terms, the movement from darkness to light for the Catholic Church in Kenya can be characterized as a conceptual and practical movement from crisis to *kairos*. Hindered by history, negative popular opinion, and ineffective education efforts, there is now renewed hope for those living with infection throughout Kenya, as religious institutions and organizations are providing both care and support for this largely silenced, marginalized, and overlooked segment of the population. This is a radical and indeed revolutionary development both theologically and practically—particularly at the grassroots level through activism and advocacy—where the Church is an active participant in the discourse on epidemiology and public health.

Catholic Church leaders acknowledge there is much work still to be done with its objectives and strategic aims regarding prevention, education, and destigmatization. And yet, AIDS remains a real problem for millions of Kenyans, one that affects all segments of the country's population. The Church as a major health-care provider, educator, activist, and religious presence in Kenyan society can move to change the hearts and minds of all Kenyans, thereby bringing about God's presence in their individual and collective activity as a *kairos* moment. This is exactly what the Catholic Church is actively called to do in providing prevention and health-care resources; to educate the population on HIV risk and susceptibility as well as treatment; and ease the stigma that those living with HIV and AIDS face in their lives so they can lead life in the fullness of Christ with their inherent human dignity and integrity intact.

It is perhaps helpful by way of conclusion to revisit the theological mandate of the Church and of those individuals working on behalf of the Church in prevention, education, and destigmatization efforts in the field, particularly at the grassroots level, "that all may have life, and have it abundantly."[152] Reformulated interrogatively, what does it mean to have life and to have life in full? From a Catholic perspective, this undoubtedly includes providing care for the physical person through health care, providing religious care for the spirit through education, sacrament, and scripture, and finally, providing intrinsic care to the human as human by upholding their dignity through programs aimed at stigma mitigation. This is true, not only of those living with infection in Nairobi, but for humans everywhere and common to all.

While not mutually exclusive, the three challenges for the Catholic Church in raising awareness of AIDS can be reframed in positive terms, using positive theology as an opportunity for *kairos*, where religious leaders attend to the human—both spiritually and physiologically—in advocating for the preferential option for those Kenyans living with HIV and AIDS, to have life and "to have it in full." Yet it remains to be seen whether these goals can be realized, not only in Kenya but throughout the rest of the world in affirming the dignity of those living with illness. Many of these obstacles—particularly the issues of sexuality, gender roles, and condom use as they pertain to AIDS prevention will be taken up in the concluding chapter.

This chapter established the parameters within which to consider the presence and activity of the Catholic Church in Kenya, particularly as this relates to a holistic, grassroots approach in responding to the AIDS epidemic in Nairobi, Kenya. By initially considering the history of the Church in East Africa as not only a religious presence but also as an important health-care provider and educator, it then proposed Fr. A. E. Orobator's binary framework of crisis and *kairos* to examine some of the challenges and opportunities facing church leaders in their efforts in prevention, education, and destigmatization. Thus, in moving from crisis to *kairos* and from despair to hope, the Catholic Church has been able to positively transform how it responds to the spiritual and physical needs of those Kenyans living with the virus.

For prevention, the initial epidemiological history presented a crisis of silence and denial, which has given way to the *kairos* or proactive treatment and programs directed to preempt future infection. In education, the crisis of disseminating incorrect information on disease origin and transmission has turned now to the *kairos* of a comprehensive curriculum developed on HIV and AIDS, supported by both religious institutions and the government. Third and finally, Catholic efforts in destigmatization have moved past the crisis of moral judgment toward modes of infection to the *kairos* of asserting and affirming that everyone—irrespective of seropositive status—deserves to be treated with basic human dignity that is never diminished in order that all humans can experience a life in which they are able to achieve their full potential.

These developments are in themselves revolutionary. The Catholic Church in its efforts is raising AIDS awareness and has moved from crisis to *kairos* theologically and practically. The Church response to the AIDS epidemic in Nairobi, therefore, must necessarily engage the human and divine realms that allows for a multi-sectorial, interdisciplinary approach to combat mistaken popular notions of the disease, ineffective educational initiatives, and biased prevention programs. In accepting the present epidemic as an actual social crisis, the Church and its clergy can realistically transform the hearts and minds of all Kenyans so that they can accept, accompany, and stand in solidarity with those infected.

The next chapter adapts largely the same structure for analyzing the Sunni Muslim response to HIV and AIDS in Kenya from a specifically Islamic perspective. Beginning with a brief overview of the history of Islam in East Africa, it then considers a case study of Muslims in Nairobi confronting HIV infection in their own religious communities. Then, as Muslim theologians, philosophers, and jurists have produced markedly fewer religious reflections on the state of the AIDS epidemic not only in Kenya but in general, I propose that the conceptual framework of crisis and *kairos* as challenge and opportunity might be useful in examining the lived, practical response of Muslim leaders in Nairobi living through and confronting daily the issues of HIV and AIDS in their own communities. In exploring raw interview data from Muslim representatives, the chapter evaluates the Muslim response to the disease in the specific areas of prevention, education, and destigmatization similar in structure to this present chapter. This then sets the stage for a theological reflection of the similarities of both the Muslim and Catholic notions of mercy, hospitality, and justice as complementary in chapter 4. Now, we will consider the Muslim response to HIV and AIDS in prevention, education, and destigmatization.

NOTES

1. Selections from the Bible are from *The New Oxford Annotated Bible: New Revised Standard Version with the Apocrypha*, ed. Michael D. Coogan (New York: Oxford University Press, 2001). The opening quotation can be found at Matthew 25:36.

2. Orobator, *From Crisis to Kairos*, 64.

3. The term *Kairos* has deep social, historical, and theological import. For example, the Kairos Document (KD) drafted by South African theologians in 1985 criticized the ecumenical response to the ongoing apartheid state. The document, "distinguishes between 'genuine reconciliation' and 'false reconciliation' by arguing that justice must accompany 'genuine reconciliation.' Justice, according to the document, should not be reduced to questions of individual guilt but should rather entail a radical change in social structure." Bronwyn Leebaw, "Legitimation or Judgment? South Africa's Restorative Approach to Transitional Justice," *Polity* 36.1 (October 2003), 34. In a similar way, the term *kairos* adapted for this project also calls for social transformation in Kenya's appointed time for God's decisive action.

4. G.S.P. Freeman-Grenville, "Vasco Da Gama's Discovery of East Africa for Portugal 1498," in *The East African Coast: Selected Documents from the First to the Earlier Nineteenth Century*, G.S.P. Freeman-Grenville, comp. (London UK: Oxford at the Clarendon Press, 1962), 50–56; Paul V. Kollman, *The Evangelization of Slaves and Catholic Origins in Eastern Africa* (Maryknoll, NY: Orbis Books, 2005), 9–22.

5. Personal Interview—Nairobi, Kenya, 6.18.14.

6. Kollman, *The Evangelization of Slaves*, 113–15.

7. Ibid., 200–204.

8. Felicitas Becker, *Becoming Muslim in Mainland Tanzania, 1890–2000* (London, UK: Oxford University Press for the British Academy, 2008), 124–27; 447–48.

9. CIA, "Africa—Kenya." This number might or might not be accurate, though the magisterial and hierarchical nature of the Church organization and leadership lend themselves to a somewhat more reliable accounting of its religious faithful.

10. Michael J. Kelly, SJ, *HIV and AIDS: A Social Justice Perspective* (Nairobi, Kenya: Paulines Publications Africa, 225.

11. Margaret A. Farley, *Compassionate Respect: A Feminist Approach to Medical Ethics and Other Questions* (Mahwah, NJ: Paulist Press, 2002), 40. For an extended discussion on the compassion as it relates to human experience, suffering, and compassion, see the author's article entitled "How Shall We Love in a Postmodern World?" *The Annual of the Society of Christian Ethics* 14 (1994): 3–19.

12. UNAIDS, *Global Report*, A7.

13. U.S. President's Emergency Plan for AIDS Relief (PEPFAR), *Kenya—Country Operational Plan—FY 2014* (Washington, DC: Office of the U.S. Global AIDS Coordinator and Health Diplomacy), 2.

14. The quotation in the subheading is a reference to the Bible, Luke 9:18.

15. While the voice of Kenyan Muslims will be explored in the subsequent chapter, certain African Islamic theologians, for example, Malik Badri from Sudan and Farid Esack from South Africa, offer diverse viewpoints on the root causes of how the virus spreads cited elsewhere in this manuscript. See Malik Badri, "The AIDS Crisis: An Islamic Perspective," in *Islam and AIDS: Between Scorn, Pity, and Justice*, eds. Farid Esack and Sarah Chiddy (Oxford, UK: Oneworld Publishing, 2009), 28–35; and Farid Esack, "Practitioner Response," in *Religion and HIV and AIDS: Charting the Terrain*, ed. Beverly Haddad (Scottsville, South Africa: University of Kwazulu-Natal Press, 2011), 213–15.

16. Laurenti Magesa, "Contextualizing HIV and AIDS in the African Reality," in *HIV and AIDS in Africa: Christian Reflection, Public Health, Social Transformation*, ed. Jacquineau Azetsop, SJ (Maryknoll, NY: Orbis Books, 2016), 19.

17. Ibid., 23.

18. Festo Mkenda, SJ, "Of Things Old and New: The African Sociohistorical Context of an HIV-and-AIDS Theology," in *HIV and AIDS in Africa: Christian Reflection, Public Health, Social Transformation*, ed. Jacquineau Azetsop, SJ (Maryknoll, NY: Orbis Books, 2016), 12.

19. Ibid., 13–14.

20. Teresia Mbari Hinga, "AIDS, Religion and Women in Africa: Theo-Ethical Challenges and Imperatives," in *Women, Religion and HIV and AIDS in Africa: Responding to Ethical and Theological Challenges*, ed. Teresia Mbari Hinga et al. (Pietermaritzburg, South Africa: Cluster Publications, 2008), 88–91.

21. Teresia Mbari Hinga, "Africa's Transformative Responses to the Gendered Global HIV and AIDS Syndemic," *HIV and AIDS in Africa: Christian Reflection, Public Health, Social Transformation*, ed. Jacquineau Azetsop, SJ (Maryknoll, NY: Orbis Books, 2016), 226.

22. Ibid., 238.

23. Self-consciously Hinga concludes, "To express this ideal, the African women theologians deliberately adopted the idea of the circle as a metaphor describing their vision of church and society. Naming themselves the "circle" signified their intention to overcome hierarchical thinking, which facilitated the use and abuse of power as domination. Ibid.

24. Ibid.

25. Domoka Lucinda Manda, "Comparative Ethics and HIV and AIDS: Interrogating the Gaps," in *Religion and HIV and AIDS: Charting the Terrain*, ed. Beverly Haddad (Scottsville, South Africa: University of Kwazulu-Natal Press, 2011), 210.

26. Kenyan Episcopal Conference (KEC), "The Church Presents Her Strategy," in *This We Teach and Do: Catholic Church and AIDS in Kenya*, Vol. 1—*Policy* (Nairobi, Kenya: Paulines Publications Africa, 2006), 35.

27. Catholic Bishops of Africa and Madagascar, "KENYA, The Challenge of AIDS," in *Speak Out on HIV & AIDS* (Nairobi, Kenya: Paulines Publications Africa, 2006), 12. A similar sentiment, that the body of Christ has AIDS can be found in Kevin Kelly, "Conclusion: A Moral Theologian Faces the New Millennium in a Time of AIDS" in *Catholic Ethicists on HIV/AIDS Prevention*, 324–32.

28. KEC, "The Church Speaks and Teaches," in *This We Teach and Do*, 29–30.

29. KEC, "Foreword," in *This We Teach and Do*, 7.

30. Pope Benedict XVI, "Healing and Forming the Whole Person" in *AIDS in Africa,* 15.

31. KEC, "The Church Presents Her Strategy," 35.

32. Ibid.

33. KEC, "The Church Speaks and Teaches," 17.

34. Michael Czerny, SJ, "Working for Healing" in *AIDS in Africa*, 52.

35. KEC, "The Church Speaks and Teaches," 20.

36. Ibid.

37. Ibid., 21.

38. Ibid.

39. Ibid.

40. KEC, "The Church Presents Her Strategy," 43.

41. Czerny, "Working for Healing," 58.

42. Orobator, "When AIDS Comes to Church,"128.

43. Ibid.

44. J. Michael McDermott, SJ, "Is AIDS God's Punishment?," *Homiletic & Pastoral Review* 32 (April 1991), 32–58.

45. Personal Interview—Nairobi, Kenya, 6.18.14.

46. Orobator, *From Crisis to Kairos*, 130.

47. Ibid., 123.

48. Pope John Paul II, "Christ, Hope for Africa—Message for the 13th World Day of the Sick," in Catholic Bishops of Africa and Madagascar, *Speak Out on HIV & AIDS*, 132.

49. Heather Snidle and David Yeoman, *Christ in AIDS: An Educational, Pastoral and Spiritual Approach to HIV/AIDS* (Cardiff, UK: Cardiff Academic Press, 1997), 36.

50. Personal Interview—Nairobi, Kenya, 6.18.14.

51. PEPFAR, *Kenya*, 4.

52. Personal Interview—Nairobi, Kenya, 6.18.14.

53. Ibid.

54. PEPFAR, *Kenya*, 2.

55. Personal Interview—Nairobi, Kenya, 7.5.14.

56. The American United Methodist theologian, Donald E. Messer, writes about this social development in *Breaking the Conspiracy of Silence: Christian Churches and the Global AIDS Crisis*, xi–xx. From a specifically Catholic perspective, Michael J. Kelly writes about silence in his work, *HIV and AIDS: A Social Justice Perspective*, 239–43.
57. Personal Interview—Nairobi, Kenya, 7.5.14.
58. Ibid.
59. Ibid.
60. Ibid.
61. Ibid.
62. *The Constitution of Kenya*, § 43.1.a.
63. Personal Interview—Nairobi, Kenya, 6.13.14.
64. Ibid.
65. Ibid.
66. Ibid.
67. Personal Interview—Nairobi, Kenya, 6.18.14.
68. Ibid.
69. Personal Interview—Nairobi, Kenya, 6.13.14.
70. Ibid.
71. Ibid.
72. Personal Interview—Nairobi, Kenya, 6.18.14.
73. Ibid.
74. Personal Interview—Nairobi, Kenya, 6.20.14.
75. Personal Interview—Nairobi, Kenya, 6.18.14.
76. Ibid.
77. Personal Interview—Nairobi, Kenya, 6.13.14.
78. Ibid.
79. Ibid.
80. Ibid.
81. Ibid.
82. Personal Interview—Nairobi, Kenya, 6.22.14.
83. Personal Interview—Nairobi, Kenya, 6.13.14.
84. Becker, *Becoming Muslim in Mainland Tanzania*, 247–48; Kollman, *The Evangelization of Slaves*, 206–7.
85. Personal Interview—Nairobi, Kenya, 6.13.14.
86. Ibid.
87. Ibid.
88. Personal Interview—Nairobi, Kenya, 6.18.14.
89. Awliya Alwy and Susanne Schech, "Ethnic Inequalities in Education in Kenya," *International Education Journal*, 5 (2), 2004: 267 (266–74).
90. Personal Interview—Nairobi, Kenya, 6.22.14.
91. Ibid.
92. Personal Interview—Nairobi, Kenya, 6.13.14.
93. Ibid.
94. PEPFAR, *Kenya*, 4; UNAIDS, *Global Report*, A48.
95. Personal Interview—Nairobi, Kenya, 6.20.14.
96. Ibid.
97. Personal Interview—Nairobi, Kenya, 6.13.14.
98. Ibid.
99. Personal Interview—Nairobi, Kenya, 6.18.14.
100. Personal Interview—Nairobi, Kenya, 6.20.14.
101. Dogmatic Constitution of the Church, *Lumen Gentium* (Vatican: the Holy See, Rome, 21 November 1965). *Lumen Gentium* or the "Dogmatic Constitution of the Church" draws on the image of the Church as a church of the people, one which resembles the very population it serves. "Since the Church is in Christ like a sacrament or as a sign and instrument both of a very closely knit union with God and of the unity of the whole human race," the document reads, the Church "desires now to unfold more fully to the faithful of the Church and to the

whole world its own inner nature and universal mission" (*LG*, § 1). Speaking with critical self-reflexivity, the document advances its mandate while also promoting the dual identity of the Church. In framing the document this way, the Church recognizes the need to acknowledge its own internal self-awareness while also promoting its universal mission of attaining fuller unity in Christ. This then allows church leaders to engage the spiritual and practical aspects of Christianity, simultaneously exploring the relationship between both the heavenly and earthly dimensions of religious practice. Dogmatic Constitution of the Church, *Lumen Gentium* (Vatican: the Holy See, Rome, 21 November 1965).

102. Personal Interview—Nairobi, Kenya, 6.20.14.
103. Ibid.
104. Personal Interview—Nairobi, Kenya, 6.18.14.
105. Ibid.
106. Personal Interview—Nairobi, Kenya, 6.13.14.
107. Bible, Proverbs 9:9.
108. Personal Interview—Nairobi, Kenya, 6.20.14.
109. Ibid.
110. Ibid.
111. Ibid.
112. Ibid.
113. Kelly, *HIV and AIDS: A Social Justice Perspective*, 129.
114. Personal Interview—Nairobi, Kenya, 6.20.14.
115. Kelly, *HIV and AIDS: A Social Justice Perspective*, 129.
116. Ibid., 128.
117. Personal Interview—Nairobi, Kenya, 6.20.14.
118. Catholic Church, *Catechism of the Catholic Church: Revised in Accordance with the Official Latin Text Promulgated by Pope John Paul II* (Vatican City, Libreria Editrice Vaticana, 1997), § 2357–59.
119. Laws of Kenya, *Penal Code of 1930*, Cap. 63 § 162–63, 15 (Nairobi, Kenya: Government Printers, rev. ed. 2012). See also Library of Congress, *Laws on Homosexuality in African Nations* (Washington, DC: The Law Library of Congress, 2014), 7.
120. Personal Interview—Nairobi, Kenya, 6.20.14.
121. Ibid.
122. Personal Interview—Nairobi, Kenya, 6.13.14.
123. Ibid.
124. Ibid.
125. Ibid.
126. Personal Interview—Nairobi, Kenya, 7.14.14.
127. Ibid.
128. Ibid.
129. Ibid.
130. Personal Interview—Nairobi, Kenya, 6.20.14.
131. Bible, John 10:10.
132. Personal Interview—Nairobi, Kenya, 6.18.14.
133. Ibid.
134. Ibid.
135. Ibid.
136. Ibid.
137. On the topic of the common good within the Catholic social teaching tradition, theologian Jacques Maritain writes: "The end of society is the good of the community, of the social body. But if the good of the social body is not understood to be a common good of human persons, just as the social body itself is a whole of human persons, this conception also would lead to other errors of a totalitarian type. The common good is neither a mere collection of private goods, nor the proper good of a whole which, like the species with respect to its individuals or the hive with respect to its bees, relates the parts to itself alone and sacrifices them to itself. It is the good human life of the multitude, of a multitude of persons, it is their communion in good living. It is therefore common to both the whole and the parts into which it

flows back and which, in turn, must benefit from it." Maritain, *The Person and the Common Good*, 50–51.

138. Ibid., 55.
139. Personal Interview—Nairobi, Kenya, 6.20.14.
140. Ibid.
141. Ibid.
142. Kelly, *HIV and AIDS: A Social Justice Perspective*, 133.
143. Personal Interview—Nairobi, Kenya, 6.20.14.
144. Ibid.
145. Ibid.
146. Ibid.
147. Ibid.
148. Ibid.
149. Kelly, *HIV and AIDS: A Social Justice Perspective*.
150. Personal Interview—Nairobi, Kenya, 7.18.14.
151. Ibid.
152. Bible, John 10:10.

Chapter Two

"Did you not know that one of my servants was sick, and you did not visit him? Did you not know that if you had visited him, you would have found Me with him?"

Muslim Responses to HIV and AIDS in Nairobi, Kenya

INTRODUCTION AND PLAN FOR THE CHAPTER

As a religious tradition, Islam maintains its own history of principled ethics regarding the treatment, care, and cure of the Muslim believer.[1] Based in the Qur'ān and *Hadith* scriptures, the lived practical response of religious leaders living in Nairobi promotes a privileged place for those ignored or overlooked by the rest of society—the poor, orphans, widows, the elderly, and the sick chief among them. Concrete expressions of social justice provide opportunities for members of the Muslim community to examine and understand the lived implications of providing care to those marginalized members in a specifically human context. In this way, the theological dimensions of Islam interact and are clarified by the historical and social dimensions of the religion.

Consequently, Muslim leaders are distinctly suited to attend to the needs of their constituent population—such as that of Nairobi, Kenya—as they address issues of a spiritual as well as a corporeal nature in the daily lives of their congregations. In this chapter, we examine the actual voices of many of these religious leaders, sheikhs, and imams helping to illuminate how the religion is practiced among the Muslims in Nairobi. Additionally, this section identifies specifics areas of Islamic activity with regard to those living with AIDS in Kenya in the collective response to human suffering in order to understand how religious and human society can provide a deeper, fuller, and clear picture of practical religious life in Kenya's capital city.

The chapter begins with a brief overview of Islam in Eastern Africa both during colonialism and after independence. Among the major themes explored are how Sunni Islam interfaces with indigenous belief systems and how Islam as a lived religion approaches and understands modernity and urbanity in the modern city of Nairobi. Next, in adapting the framework from the previous chapter, the next three sections present the conceptual and practical movement from crisis to *kairos* in the identified fields of prevention, education, and destigmatization in the words of Islamic leaders living and providing care to those persons infected in Kenya's capital.

A BRIEF HISTORY OF ISLAM IN EASTERN AFRICA

To provide historical and social context, this section offers an overview of Islam in Kenya during colonialism, which serves to explain the importance of the religion geographically, as well as how Islamic practice has changed over the past five hundred years. Similar to Catholicism, Muslim charities established and funded countless schools (Arabic, *madrasa*), hospitals, and aid organizations through the centuries, thereby inhabiting an influential position both religiously and socially in the lives of Kenyan Muslims. The subsequent section provides a consideration of how the Muslim population faces the challenges of living in the cosmopolitan, ethnically-diverse, and religious pluralistic city of Nairobi.

However, to begin, we must consider the introduction and historical spread of Islam along the Swahili Coast from the fifteenth century until now. This involves a critical examination of some of the major cultural, social, and ethnic hybridization that has occurred over the past five hundred years while also considering the profound exchange of Islam and indigenous belief over this period of time.

Precolonial Islam and the Swahili Coast

Similar to Christianity, Islam has long-standing roots in Eastern Africa. Beginning as early as the ninth century, Islamic merchant sailors from the Hahdramaut region of Oman began trading with the indigenous Africans of the continent's Swahili Coast along the Indian Ocean.[2] The cultural exchange included far more than just goods, as the traders from Shiraz set up a sultanate along the archipelago of islands off the coast of present-day Tanzania and Kenya.[3] Intermarriage created a distinct Swahili ethnic identity, mixing Arab and indigenous African elements while the slave trade and exchange of exotic African goods to the Arabian Peninsula insured that those sultanates established in Kilwa Kisiwani, Lamu, and Zanzibar would endure for centuries.[4]

Even with this interaction and exchange with the mainland, Islam continued to gain prominence throughout the islands off the East African Coast after the Sultan of Oman, Sayid Said Ibn Sultan (d. 1870), moved his sultanate to Zanzibar in the early 1800's with trade continuing to increase between the island regions well into the twentieth century.[5] Major commodities included ivory, tortoise shell, rubber, and above all slaves who left the coastal towns such as Mombasa and Bagamoyo in present day Kenya and Tanzania to be bought and sold in Stone Town on Zanzibar Island.[6]

By the end of the nineteenth century with the interventions of German and British colonizing influences, the slave trade all but collapsed and the Sultan of Oman opened Zanzibar to French, German, American, and British exporters.[7] Then, in 1895, the British Crown claimed a protectorate over much of mainland East Africa, including the Great Rift Valley as far west as Lake Naivasha.[8] This was later extended to Uganda in 1902 in what was then referred to the British East African Protectorate.[9] With their superior firearms and sense for infrastructure, the British colonial administration was able to quell any indigenous uprising and brought much of East Africa—all the way to the Swahili Coast—under British rule. Thus, by 1920, the Crown formally announced the British East African Protectorate as a colony of the Crown and British commercial interests continued to spread throughout the mainland.

However, though the Muslims were well-versed in administrative and bookkeeping skills, the British colonial authorities preferred the coastal Bantu tribes who they believed they could civilize and whose souls they could save through the life-giving message of Christianity.[10] As an interesting sociohistorical development, under British rule the Swahili Muslims were relatively free through the British policy of indirect rule to practice their religion. However Christianity among the Muslim community was considered to be the religion of the colonizers. Thus, in the early twentieth century, Islam continued to spread fastest even as Arab rule in Zanzibar was ending, in part because the religion was seen by many indigenous Africans as a subversive political reaction to colonization.[11]

With the demise of the slave trade and the resulting diminished political and economic power of the Sultanate between 1880 and 1920, the office of sultan became a largely ceremonial position and Arab Islam began to lose its once prominent position along the Swahili Coast.[12] Yet certain factions of indigenous Islam such as Qadiriyya and Alawiyya Sufism continued to gain popularity throughout Eastern Africa due to its view as an inclusive and egalitarian religion.[13] During this period of colonization, Islamic religious authority was renegotiated in light of colonization and the British administration's power and influence, even as the term "Muslim" was used loosely and adopted a very fluid definition. There were the Omani Arabs of Shirazi descent of the island archipelago; the itinerant Sufi imams who would travel from village to village spreading the message of Islam further and further into the mainland; there were the Bantu converts to Islam who continued to practice their indigenous religion; numerous Shi'i East Asian Muslim traders and rail workers transplanted their lives and families to East Africa; and there were those who were Muslim in name only—those who did not practice Islamic devotional life but converted for economic benefits or educational opportunities. This is but a small sampling of the number of Islamic factions that arose historically throughout Kenya even up to the country's independence from Britain in 1964.

Islam in Postindependence Kenya

After independence in 1964, the British left the daily infrastructural workings up to the local people, which created a vacuum of authority and leadership.[14] This also led to a tense relationship between the predominately Christian Bantu and the Swahili Muslims in the newly independent state, notably in the field of education which was adapted from the British Christian-based curriculum.[15] Where Christian schools had been historically established and funded by the colonial administration during British rule, these schools continued to be funded by the government of Kenya's first president, Jomo Kenyatta—a Christian Kikuyu.[16]

However, the Islamic schools were left to meet the local needs of the country's Muslim population unfunded by the government. These locally supported Islamic educational organizations displayed characteristics markedly different from the British mission schools, in that the Muslim teachers worked with the local authorities to gradually develop a curriculum of religious teaching practices instead of advocating and supporting a foreign, Christian structure of education.[17] Especially since the imams came from the local villages, they maintained a certain pride in the self-sufficiency of this educational model even though it did raise some methodological issues such as the consistency of content and effective instruction.[18]

Additionally, because of the decentralized nature of Islamic teaching, religious practitioners saw themselves as Muslim by virtue of praying in a Muslim fashion and not necessarily being based in religious scholarship. In the words of one Muslim living in postcolonial Eastern Africa, he described himself "as a Muslim *wa kusali tu*, 'who just prays,' as opposed to one who has studied the Quran."[19] Those Muslims who wanted to pursue higher education in this period of post-British independence would have to travel from their villages to other Islamic lands such as Zanzibar, off the coast of Tanzania, and Mombasa in Kenya, or even to the Middle East for educational opportunities past primary school. Local religious authorities on the other hand were left to spread Islamic teaching by themselves and, as a result, Islamic ritual was taught and practiced inconsistently throughout this coastal region. Particularly in the realm of Islamic law, a major area of education and teaching, "the application of Islamic law remained haphazard. Changes in domestic and family relationships were not unrelated to Islamic law, but neither did they correspond to its letter. The most influential element of Muslim teachings in these ongoing negotiations probably was general, often implicit value judgments, rather than specific rules."[20]

Over time, this trend changed how the religion was understood from the city to the rural countryside with serious students often migrating to centers of Islamic education, leading to a conceptual shift in terms of how Islam was taught in the cities as well as in the rural, cultural imagination of the religion. In the subsequent objectification and fragmentation of Islam, this historical shift in the rural perception of the religion coincided with "the distinction between public and private sphere, which was justified to appeal to Islam. Like the distinction between town and countryside, it was an ideological definition applied to very variable practical realities."[21]

During this time, a disconnect arose between Islamic teaching in the countryside and the cities:

> The dividing line between ideologies born in the African environments of the towns and the imported varieties followed the economic and vocational distinctions between the coastal towns and the *nyika* [bush region found just outside of the villages]. Among *walimu* [elder teachers], some specialized in sciences which borrowed more from imported wisdom, while others' learning came from the accumulated wisdom of the town's *bara* [mainland areas across from or behind the Swahili town]. Thus, there arose a rough distinction between "town" learning (*elimu*) and "bush" learning (*uganga*). (However, many *walimu* were known to be *waganga*. It was *uganga* which was thought to be non-religious, while *elimu* was "religion," properly speaking, to townspeople even though *elimu* itself included much that was African.) Town learning was considered religion, while knowledge which came from non-Islamic regions adjacent to the coast simply was "medicine."[22]

For example, where the insistence on Qur'ānic memorization was the mainstay of local *madrasa* teaching, Qur'ānic exegesis (Arabic, *tafsir*) was not stressed and Arabic was generally not taught or practiced with competent Arabic speakers.[23] This development has historically led to a very superficial understanding of the Qur'ān among contemporary coastal Muslims, and the decentralized educational structure where local congregations followed the teachings of one specific imam led to diverse interpretations of the religion.

One other notable aspect of the adaptive nature of Islam in Eastern Africa is that, because of religious pluralism in general, Islamic devotional practice along the Swahili Coast during this period of postcolonial independence began to assimilate certain indigenous practices and elements. Certainly, Islam and Christianity are relatively new religious traditions to the African subcontinent when compared to the much older indigenous religious traditions that have been practiced for centuries prior, resulting to a unique mixture of foundational Islamic teaching and indigenous practices.

ISLAM AND INDIGENOUS RELIGIOUS TRADITIONS

Even as Islam began to spread farther into the mainland, many villages held tight to their traditional beliefs and practices and, among the Bantu tribes of the hinterlands, "until recently very few were Muslims; most respected the spirits of their own particular lineage and clan ancestors."[24] In many cases, Islam was conceptually compatible with certain religious structures—among them those that stressed humility, self-control, charity, chastity, and the promotion of the common good of the community over the individual—strikingly similar to its Christian social justice counterpart.

Specifically among these traditional widespread beliefs are the traditional cult of ancestor worship and belief in sorcery. While certainly not recognized as a legitimate form of worship among educated East African Muslim leaders, they differ in the extent to which these practices affect Islamic self-understanding. In fact, among the Islamic leaders interviewed for this project, one claimed that venerating ancestors was *shirk*—the Islamic sin of worshipping gods other than God—while another acknowledged that this practice does in fact happen.[25] Throughout Nairobi, locals still perform ceremonies associated with ancestor worship, even though the ritual fundamentally conflicts with foundational notions of being an avowed Muslim.

With ancestor worship, the indigenous belief structure gives rise to recommended models of behavior for local populations on how to live one's life—not unlike the Islamic concept of *taqlid* or "imitation" based on the lives and legacies of certain pious individuals who have gone before in the family lineage. In this way, ancestor worship is not innovation (Arabic, *bid'a*) but given the open framework of African indigenous practice, the rituals can be seen to complement Muslim self-identification:

> The way individuals interpreted relationships with ancestors and spirits, and increasingly with god, mattered because it defined their options in interacting with the spirit world, hence in enhancing and safeguarding their lives. Nevertheless, as long as being a Muslim and interacting with the spirit world were considered compatible, being a Muslim could be thought of as a way of *improving*, not renouncing, previously known religious practices. Religious

> change, in this sense, can be described as part of a search for ways to improve life. It need not be motivated by disenchantment with existing ways, but it implies an admission that things could be better.[26]

While the practice varies from village to village and from culture to culture, one common theme can be seen as humanity participating in the continuum of birth, life, and death. However, with such a variation in actual practice, Islamic teachings interfaced and in some ways adapted to local culture resulting in often drastically different views on the veneration of ancestors.

This exchange of culture and religious understanding created a highly complex and socially conditioned sense of being Muslim in postcolonial Kenya, not only along the coastal region but also in areas more distant into the mainland and in cities such as Nairobi. As this interchange pertains to ancestor worship, the dead are not dead insofar as they can still communicate and interact in the lives of the living and those not yet born, both for purposes of good and bad.[27] Consequently, the ancestors, overwhelmingly male in keeping with the increased gendering of Islam during this period in history, are paragons of virtue even after their death.[28] These ancestors must die of natural causes—violent deaths and deaths associated with sexual immorality such as HIV and AIDS precludes one from attaining ancestor status—and the ancestor must leave behind male progeny who will continue his memory as well as his legacy of virtue. Altars to these individuals are kept in households throughout Eastern Africa, and on special feast days, sacrifices of money, food, and even of alcohol—though forbidden in Islam—are made to those ancestors to insure good fortune or for supplication if misfortune has befallen a member of the family.[29]

In a notable adaptation of this practice as a way of imploring spiritual intercessors to act on behalf of the supplicant, Islamic leaders from the villages within which they serve as imams and sheikhs operate with the succinct formulation, " 'do not worship/pray to objects or trees,' *msiabudu vitu* or *miti*, or more subtly, 'do not worship *via* objects,' *msiabudu kupitia vitu*." To worship "through" things would be a form of *shirk*, attributing partners to God. Rather, by cleverly adapting indigenous practice to Islamic teachings, "Muslim prayers offered the alternative to 'praying through things.' The expression 'to pray through things' itself, though, allowed for the possibility that the prayers were directed to the right place, if by the wrong means. It was less dismissive of local practice than the claim that it consisted in 'praying to things.' "[30] In other words, instead of praying to other things for help in the physical world, these believers could complement their belief in Islam with intercessory prayers through things that still affirm the Islamic principle of *tawhīd*, or the "unicity" of God. Though ancestor worship venerated those who had gone before as members of the spiritual world, the question remains if it is licit in Islam to consult those living for questions related to their lives, family, and property outside of the learned hierarchy of Muslim leadership. For this, we now turn to a discussion of Islam and sorcery.

Sorcery and Islam in Coastal Kenya

One other area of indigenous worship that has influenced contemporary Islamic practice in coastal Eastern Africa—practically if not conceptually—is the belief in sorcery and the power of divinatory practitioners. The ability to communicate with the spiritual world, termed *uganga* in KiSwahili, while outside of official Islamic teaching in rural communities, is integral in restoring social order. In the rural context, it is "the body of practice that draws upon mechanistic devices and spirit possession for divining and upon distinct patterns of ritual healing."[31] The diviners themselves, known as *mganga* (s.)/ *uganga* (pl.) serve a cathartic position within the community—once again, outside of officially sanctioned Islamic rites and practices. Among one ethnic group in Kenya, the Giriama, "Divination and healing are frequently sought by those dispossessed of work, money, land, or good health as alternatives or complements to secular efforts to improve their lot; the practitioners of divination and healing are the *aganga*."[32]

Even though these diviners complement Islamic practice in Eastern Africa, foundational Islamic belief prohibits associating anything with God. This gives rise to a creative tension with the local belief in the spirit world, manifesting itself in multiple forms—not least of all deities and ancestors. To pursue remedies from the *mganga*, then, is to seemingly commit the sin of associating another partner with God in Islam. The question therefore becomes one of the degree of infraction, since "Muslims do not dismiss the notion of spirits altogether, they treated them as a part of God's created universe."[33] Since coastal Muslims do, in fact, acknowledge the presence of spirits in the created world, it is not explicitly forbidden to offer these spiritual entities sacrifices or to communicate with them. Rather, "the problem was how to know how to do so without breaking the prohibition against *shirk*, the worshipping of gods other than God."[34] The major theological issue then becomes to what degree consulting *uganga* or making sacrifices to ancestors was acceptable under the belief structures of Islam:

> One way to think about the problem was as a matter of the right degree, of how to respect and interact with spirit forces without detracting from the adoration owed to God. But there was also concern about the ambiguous moral status of the spirit world itself, and about the possibility of exploiting interaction with it for immoral aims. Besides the danger of *shirk*, new Muslims faced the moral ambiguity both of the process of dealing with the spirit world and of the spirit world itself. This uneasiness was not new.[35]

Again, one area of concern for those who consult the *mganga* or worship at altars dedicated to their ancestors is how the current misfortune they experience had been caused in the first place. For the Muslim leader dealing with the belief in sorcery and spirit divination, the "problem was to distinguish between prohibited [Kiswahili, *haramu*] and permitted [KiSwahili, *halali*] ways of healing."[36] Indeed, many Islamic religious authorities dismissed traditional practice as purely local and, by definition, not religious. Therefore, "if it was not 'religion' it was not in competition with Muslim practice."[37]

Particularly since traditional indigenous belief was not codified by the *uganga*, it was susceptible to change and synthesizing elements from other religions, including prominently Islamic ritual and practice. Even today, many coastal Swahili diviners "incorporate objects and agents from the Muslim side into their rituals."[38] Among these elements borrowed by *uganga* are Islamic texts, most notably the Qur'ān to which some attribute talismanic healing properties. "Diviners and healers alike propitiate both Allah (sometimes referred to in Kiswahili as *Mwenje-ezi Mungu*) and Muslim spirits, using the Quran, rosewater, food such as honey, and coins and other metal objects," writes Janet McIntosh, a prominent ethnographer at Brandeis University who studies coastal Islamic communities. In an account of this religious adaptation and reflecting on the significance of the Qur'ān in Islamic devotional life, "Healers may prepare talismans and treatments containing scraps of the Quran and Arabic writing, while diviners may call upon possessing Muslim spirits to help them 'read' and 'write' the Quran."[39]

A final note on spirit divination and its interface with Islam: Muslims who choose to consult *uganga* instead of Islamic officials may do so because of social and cultural sensibilities. However, this dynamic between traditional and official religion also highlights the tension between rural and urban life regarding ideas associated with health and healing. In the local understanding of social catharsis informed by agrarian communitarianism peculiar to farming villages throughout Kenya, the *uganga* is necessary for the townspeople to coexist, since the belief in spirit divination influences Islamic practice instead of taking away from it, particularly in situations where formal Islamic teaching might be unclear. Once more, in Eastern African coastal Muslim communities, there is widespread belief that spirits do exist as part of God's created universe. Consulting the local *mganga* could then be considered to be entirely consistent with the Qur'ān as well as helpful and licit (*halali*) in the daily lives of these Muslims as a matter of social cohesion.

The root cause of the problems experienced in these villages, however, may have a social, communal dimension in the previously cited continuum between birth, life, and death. This is mainly because, "to the mind of practitioners of local religion, too, spirits, and those who dealt with them, held the power both to protect and to harm. This was a practical problem, since the interaction with spirits and ancestors mattered in everyday life."[40] While not officially recognized or sanctioned by Islamic religious authorities, those who could communicate with the spirit world held some practical power in the everyday life of coastal Muslims. Even among some educated individuals, the *uganga* "were essential to healing, and more broadly to the safeguarding of individuals, households, and villages. The interaction of jealous or neglected ancestral spirits was, and to some extent still is, considered the likely reason for many misfortunes."[41]

The *Uchawi* and Other Negative Social Manifestations

In making the conceptual link between the health and well-being of the individual and that of the community, spirit divination is a practice that has its roots in precolonial and pre-Islamic East Africa, particularly among the Swahili Coast. In order to make sense of misfortune, the believer—whether they be self-identified Catholic or Muslim—will attempt to placate these ancestral spirits, which remains essential in keeping people and the community functioning properly. By reinforcing this social structure of interaction with the spirit world, a special focus was given those individuals who are viewed as being able to conjure unnatural powers to negatively influence other members of the community.

These outsiders, referred to in KiSwahili as *mchai* (s.)/*uchawi* (pl.) for "witch" or "sorcerer" are often considered as a malevolent recluse who can be vanquished through certain ritual and often communally cathartic processes.[42] The *uganga* are instrumental in these rites since "spirit forces were involved in dealing with witchcraft, and it would have been hard to address witchcraft fears without consulting healers who knew how to interact with the spirits."[43] Yet consulting the diviners on matters of witchcraft could create a tense relationship between the spirit world and its influence on Islamic practice, especially when the use of medicine—both Western and indigenous—was added to the equation. Learned Islamic practice as a prescribed lifestyle maintains a generally open and favorable view of health care and medicine, with *Hadith* traditions stating, "God has sent down both the disease and the cure, and He has appointed a cure for every disease, so treat yourselves medically, but use nothing unlawful."[44]

This last prohibition, to refrain from using anything that violates the religious restrictions of Islam, becomes a rather grey area when consulting traditional healers, since the *uganga* can prescribe a particular medicine for the client. This regimen might be religiously problematic for Islam since the medicines themselves "derived their strength from the spirit world, or because using their powers meant interfering with the order of things intended by God."[45] The Muslim religious authorities were then faced with a practical dilemma. Instead of explicitly stating that the medicines produced by the spirit diviners did not work and were not licit in Islam, religious officials strove to have people reformulate their ideas pertaining to indigenous medicine in ways compatible with their belief in the Islamic principle of *tawhīd*, God's unicity. Health care—of the individual and the community; local and urban; real and perceived; Islamic or traditional—has thus long been a topic of discussion for those Muslims living along the Swahili Coast in renegotiating ideas associated with the corporeal body in light of social, cultural, and even geographic influences.

To conclude, historically the interaction between the Omani Sultanate and the British colonial conquest of the region by the British East African Company created a highly nuanced Islamic self-identity. As a direct result, the educational system of Kenya clearly exhibits the creative tension among contemporary Muslims regarding their religious, cultural, and ethnic realities. Yet, a fascinating development is the inclusion of certain indigenous belief systems within Muslim communities along the Swahili Coast. These practices—specifically ancestor worship and belief in the power of spirit divination—indicates a specifically Eastern African coastal Islamic identity that has developed gradually throughout the centuries in ways unique to this complex social milieu and geographic location.

KENYAN ISLAM IN A MODERN CONTEXT

Where the previous section considered the history of Islam and the adaptation and incorporation of indigenous elements into mainstream religious practice, this section offers some examination and insight into how Islam has articulated its own voice in the discourse of modernity and postcolonialism specific to East Africa. To begin, we must acknowledge that there is not one "Islam" but many different iterations and formulations of the tradition. In effect, this yields an ongoing process of constructing an Islamic identity that at once reflects local context while also being influenced by more foundational teachings.

Take, for example, Kenya. Muslims in the East African country represent a religious minority with some estimates at between 8 and 11 percent of the country's population, while other sources place this estimate closer to 33 percent.[46] Of this, the overwhelming majority of these are Sunni Muslim of Swahili and indigenous African descent, yet there are also Muslims of Southeast Asian and Arab ethnicity. Though the largest ethnic group in Kenya is the Kikuyu (at 22 percent), the capital city boasts communities of each of Kenya's numerous ethnic and religious groups making it all but impossible to identify one specific ethnic Islamic identity. Among Shi'i, the Ithna-Ashari, Ahmadiyya, as well as Nizari-Ismailyya communities can be found throughout the country.[47] From my fieldwork and according to my informants, it would seem as though there is little in the way of tension between the different ethnicities, between Muslims and non-Muslims, and even between the different factions of Islam in Nairobi. All of the subjects interviewed were Sunni, and so the current research leaves out an important voice, that of Shi'i Islam which is a methodological limitation. However, as the Sunni Muslims represent the majority, it would reason that these views presented here are general and widely held.

The remainder of this chapter proceeds in this way. Having conducted field research in Nairobi, the next three sections consider the lived response of Sunni Muslim leaders who live and work in the city to HIV and AIDS using their own words. Since these leaders inhabit a specific social and historical context, there exists an intriguing overlap between theology and lived religious practice. Again, similar in structure to the Catholic voice analyzed in the previous chapter, this structure proposes a dichotomy for Islamic authority in prevention, education and destigmatization in that all three represent not only a crisis for the Islamic community of Nairobi, but they also represent an opportunity (or *kairos* to use the Christian terminology) to face the current epidemic in Kenya as leaders of an important faith community. The chapter now considers the response of Muslims in Nairobi to HIV prevention as crisis.

PREVENTION AS CRISIS

"Yes, this disease could be viewed from a historical perspective. In the initial stages, Muslims considered HIV as a disease that affects the immoral society and considered it more of immorality rather than a disease. And they considered it as a punishment from God for the wrongdoings of the human society," stated one Muslim doctor working in the field of health care. "And this is a belief that is confirmed by the teachings of Islam, that if people become promiscuous and they don't care about their morality then diseases like this would come. So the response was that anybody who got infected with HIV would be somebody who deserves that punishment because of their own doings. So this is the historical thing."[48]

This observation identifies one of the largest issues facing prevention initiatives among the Muslim population—that of moralistic judgment regarding people living with HIV infection. One prominent dimension of this moralization of the virus lies in the continued process of renegotiating Islamic identity in the face of urbanity and modernity in Nairobi. Where historically, the individual Muslim was tied to the local, organic community in the coastal Swahili regions, the movement to urban centers forced religious groups to redefine what it means to be a Muslim in contemporary Nairobi. Most notably, the purification or reformulation of Islamic identity in the face of modernity has been largely influenced in Eastern Africa by such leaders as Sheikh Al-Amin Al-Mazrui (d. 1947) and Sheikh Abdallah Saleh Al-Farsy (d. 1982) who themselves were associated with reformist theologies throughout other parts of the Islamic world.[49]

Thus, when it comes to HIV and AIDS prevention, the Muslim community in Nairobi—similar in many ways to the Catholic reaction—perceive that the disease is associated with people who had engaged in immoral or religiously illicit behavior, including those that accepted modernity and allowed for an upheaval of the social order.[50] This is due in large part to the belief that HIV was not a Muslim problem. Said one imam who preaches at a central mosque in downtown Nairobi, "I can also say that it has not really—HIV and AIDS—has not been institutionalized within the Muslim community, within the Muslim structures. If it is institutionalized, then it will be easy for us to intervene because we will own the process. It is—HIV and AIDS programs are still owned by other people, and not by the [Muslim] community."[51]

This other-izing view of the disease among Kenyan Muslims makes strategic objectives for prevention difficult to establish and even more difficult to maintain. Reformulating Islamic practice in light of modernity and urbanity in Nairobi has proven troublesome since, on the one hand an acceptance or ownership of HIV and AIDS as an Islamic problem might prove scandalous to religious interpretations of sexuality and immorality; while on the other hand, denying that the epidemic exists serves to create an atmosphere of denial and silence which can threaten to worsen an already tense situation. While this dynamic will be analyzed in a less positive, comparative light in chapter 4, the very nature of Nairobi as Kenya's capital city demands that residents negotiate a complex web of cultural, ethnic, social, economic, political, and not least of all, religious identities.

When confronted with urbanity and modernity, living in the city poses a distinct challenge for Kenyan Muslims, particularly in terms of what is deemed acceptable behavior. Observed one other imam working in the field of health care and prevention, "Nairobi is a metropolitan city, whereby you get everybody coming from everywhere and going out from everywhere. You get people of different attitudes, practices, behaviors and so on so forth. Nairobi is a place where drugs are there. There are a lot of issues being a big city."[52] As the largest urban center in Kenya with a population of over three million people, Nairobi is a city where the exchange of ideas and cultures is a constant and ongoing process.[53] Remarking on the conceptual shift from city to village life, the imam continued, "you can compare it with a small village, whereby you know everything is centralized, people are living the same as one community and so on so forth. So I think because of so many factors, it wouldn't be surprising to see Nairobi different from other towns."[54]

Representative of this description, instead of stressing the communal nature of the coastal village life where people live as "one community," this interlocutor emphasizes that Nairobi is drastically different than rural life where everything is decentralized. Maintaining a unique sense of Islamic identity, then, may be difficult in the face of religious, ethnic, and cultural diversity, especially as this relates to preventing the spread of HIV. On further reflection, keeping a consistent interpretation of Islamic teaching might additionally prove difficult, particularly when coupled with the myriad challenges and temptations of city life. On this topic, the imam concludes, "issues like—ok—for example, drugs. Drugs not in the sense of only hard drugs, cocaine and so on so forth . . . heroin. Even these illicit brew of which last month, I don't know if you heard, more than forty people died in one place, and another at thirty-six, and so on so forth. You see, so all these factors put together—it wouldn't be surprising that Nairobi is a bit different from other cities."[55]

The illicit brew this Muslim official mentions above is an illegal operation throughout Kenya that produces alcoholic beverages from any number of ingredients without any quality control or governmental oversight.[56] The presence of cocaine, heroin, and this illicit brew is not exclusive to Nairobi, as drug use is on the rise in coastal cities such as Lamu and Kisumu as well.[57] However, the fact that these substances are associated with urban centers is notable since it marks a shift in how Muslims view life in the city, and why prevention efforts might be hindered by the Muslim population's refusal to accept modernity—including the temptations and pitfalls present in Nairobi.

According to another Islamic public health official, intravenous drug use (IDU) is actually "on the increase because currently we have an estimation of about between 30,000 and 40,000 in the coastal area, in parts of the urban centers who are on drugs—on the hard drugs. And we feel like, according to KAIS [the Kenyan AIDS Indicator Survey], about 3.8 percent of HIV transmission in Kenya is through the drug use. And this is on the increase, definitely."[58] With over thirty thousand people on hard drugs in this subject's estimation, it is worth considering that the other-izing attitudes toward IDU's and the silence and shame associated with those addicted—in addition to the fact that needle sharing is a channel for disease transmission—explain one alarming factor in the continued spread of HIV.

Internally, as a crisis that Muslim communities in Kenya have had to confront in their daily lives, the AIDS epidemic demands that religious leaders take seriously prevention efforts as a matter of urgency. To deny that it is a Muslim problem is to overlook the very roots of the epidemic as well as the structural reasons for why it continues to spread, irrespective of religious self-identification. Prevention is hugely important since one of the major reasons for the persistence of HIV, according to one imam, goes back to the moral judgment of how the disease was contracted, stemming from immorality and a lack of values from our parents and leaders. "Now, before our fathers used to tell us that they were being guided from a young age until they were getting married," he attested. "But nowadays when a child reaches 15, we tend to believe now he is free to go to do everything that he wants. So there is immorality, poverty, lack of clear guidance from our leaders and families."[59]

With this observation, there is a very intriguing shift in focus from the agency and morality of those members of the Muslim community who are living with infection to the communal responsibility of religious leaders and parents who should teach their children the risks of contracting the disease. Though the topic of AIDS education as both a challenge and an opportunity, as will be discussed in the following section, this change in perspective makes for a notable religious development regarding the HIV crisis in that this Islamic official calls on other Muslim leaders, parents, and adults to reconsider their positions on the topic of prevention in order to provide guidance for those at-risk of contracting the infection.

Thus, one of the major obstacles facing effective prevention efforts in Nairobi is one of leadership. To speak of the "official" Muslim response to AIDS in the city can be problematic since specific imams may have drastically different views about the disease, its methods of transmission, and its etiology, which can lead to a further entrenched crisis. For one representative from the Kenyan Council of Imams (KCI), even if there is a proactive policy directed at prevention advocated by Islamic leaders, the implementation might still be problematic. "So we have developed certain positions and response mechanisms. However, in terms of how that can be implemented is still a problem. It's just an ideal situation, a dream that we have," this imam confided. "But implementation is a problem because of lack of resources. Of course we know that individual groups are doing quite a lot within the community. But unlike, you see the way the Christian community is structured—especially the Catholics or the Anglicans—they have a structure all the way from up, down. Islam doesn't have that."[60]

Navigating the waters of religious leadership and authority, this subject problematizes the position of imams speaking about HIV and AIDS prevention with the Catholic Church's magisterium since there is no one, monolithic, authoritative voice on the effects of the epidemic on the Muslim population. The imam did, however, cite the authority and presence of one of the legislative bodies operating in Nairobi, the Supreme Council of Kenyan Muslims (SUPKEM). Yet even this organization has its limitations. "So the Supreme Council of Kenya Muslims is a semblance of that [Catholic Church magisterium], but the chairman of the Supreme Council of Kenya Muslims is not a *mufti*, neither has he the authority to tell the imams what to do," he stated. "Maybe the imam's council can issue a *fatwa*, for example, on certain positions that can influence a few imams and a few Muslims, a good number of Muslims and a good number of imams. But the Supreme Council of Kenya Muslims is an honorable body, but it doesn't have impact."[61]

This critical self-assessment on structure of authority in the Islamic community has certainly made prevention efforts in Nairobi and more broadly throughout Kenya significantly more difficult. The lack of authority, initiative, or cohesive message of Muslims toward AIDS and those currently infected with the virus has done little to address the present epidemic in terms of prevention. In a severe estimation of the impact of the local imams on changing how people understand the transmission of HIV and how they treat people who are HIV positive, this imam attested, "Because of lack of that impact, even if they came up with a good policy, beautiful policy, they cannot have people implement it unless they have sensitization, advocacy, and all that." He continues, "Maybe the Kenya Council of Imams can by asking their followers, the imams, to implement it on the ground. But that's, of course, where it will end. The imam will talk about it and that is it. The community will not feel compelled to do anything. So that's a challenge."[62] Those Muslim leaders working in the field of disease prevention are thus faced with a crisis of what to do effectively to meet the needs of the Islamic population of Kenya's capital city. Similar to their Catholic counterparts, these religious officials are presented with the challenge to be agents of empowerment within their own communities, which involves changing the hearts and minds of their fellow Muslims regarding HIV and AIDS infection in Nairobi. Another respondent identified the governmental response and its use of resources as a major obstacle associated with the AIDS crisis in Kenya. In the words of one imam regarding how to prevent future infection, "I think our government does not use religious men. Because if you use religious men, you will reach that grassroots level. Yeah, [the government] makes mistakes. You see, mostly they use these artists, musicians, or wherever they go. But religious leaders are not there. If they are, they are not to the level that they should be used. If they are being used, it is not to the level that they should be used."[63] The significance and visibility of religious leadership is then held in tension with the efforts of the government in AIDS prevention for this Islamic leader.

The reason behind this disconnect between the government and the Muslim objectives in preventing future infection is that people "tend to believe more in their religious leaders than anyone else. Because people put their trust in their religious leaders more than ever—some trust them even more than they trust their own parents. So I think that if you use a religious leader to spread across, it will be more effective than using anyone else. Because they believe more in them, they have trust in them more than anyone else."[64] The Muslim leadership in Nairobi therefore has considerable influence since religious officials occupy a theologically impactful position within the community—though this impact can be either positive or negative depending on the message regarding HIV and AIDS infection being espoused.

Moving now to the government aims at disease prevention, from an Islamic perspective the major factors that have led to the AIDS crisis in Kenya can be attributed partly in terms of ineffective initiatives and partially to a lack of resources. Within the government initiatives, those Muslim leaders interviewed for this project identified a basic discrepancy between the government response to intravenous drug use, for example, and the Muslim response. "Sometimes we have differences, like in HIV control with drug-users—the government policy is on harm reduction. Muslims differed on this, where they have the exchange program for syringes and needles," admitted one sheikh on the disconnect between the government and Islamic efforts at prevention. "We felt that this did not need to go that way. We needed to address the source problem of the drugs and so on. So we don't need to address superficial issues of harm reduction when drug and substance abuse are still encouraged, the government doesn't do anything."[65]

The public perception of the importance of governmental and religious officials is an interesting distinction since at the heart of the discussion is the issue of legitimacy and whose voice really resonates with the people. Even in terms of advocacy, Islamic leaders are pivotal in pushing for social change, even when the government is unable or unwilling to act. The sheikh continued, "So we feel like the government needs to do more in stopping this issue of drugs. And we feel the issue of governance and corruption and things like that play a role in this increasing trend."[66] Interestingly, this criticism focuses in large part on the government and its failure regarding assimilation of popular culture into its response to HIV and AIDS prevention.

Another area of contention between the Muslims of Nairobi and the government involves the allocation of resources and budgetary constraints in curbing future infections. On the topic of the budget, one Muslim health official gauged the government response as initially favorable, until the topic of resources came up:

> I think the government is doing a good job. It's trying. But then, some of the issues—we don't always agree with the government. For example, today the budget is going to be read. And everybody's waiting to see how much the government is putting in. You see, what we are saying is that the private sector and the foreign donors—their response is so much bigger than our own government. So those are some of the issues which we have been telling the government. That, no, you have to show commitment. Commitment is how much you spend on those issues. So in terms of the budget, and we are waiting for the budget to be read today. But I don't think they've put a lot of money in HIV and AIDS. Although they have, but in comparison from—so we are depending on donor funding, everything donor funding. Everything donor funding.[67]

This acknowledgment that the government could be doing more in the field of prevention is noteworthy since resources for HIV prevention are becoming harder to secure. In a concluding estimation, the official reflected, "I think that effort still has to be put in. Because when you lag behind . . . the infection also comes. So I believe it should be a continuous process."[68]

This is not an uncommon sentiment, that the resources made available to HIV prevention are not a constant since they depend on international donors for support. Remarking on the balance the government must strike in terms of disease prevention, yet another Islamic scholar signaled:

> What I know is that the fact that they declared this as a national pandemic was good—as a national disaster was very good for people to seriously respond. Maybe the resources that the government has put in is not adequate. So basically, I would say on the government part, it's the resources—the inadequacy in resources. The response I think we've seen a lot of commercials on HIV and AIDS. Whether it's through government or non-governmental organizations, I really don't know. But what I know is that I've visited a few government hospitals and you find notices on HIV and AIDS. And maybe recently, the government—the political arm of the government—is not talking about HIV and AIDS because it is no longer maybe a priority. That could be an issue for me. But in terms of response, I think at the beginning we did very well, the leadership—the political leadership—used to talk about it. There was specific body formed and marketed to design programs that intervene on HIV and AIDS. So basically I think it is just resources.[69]

The above account does an admirable job in highlighting the Islamic estimation of government initiatives and the major hurdles that still exist in facing the crisis that still exists in AIDS prevention in Nairobi—that HIV is not really considered a priority among the political leadership and thus Islamic leaders need to address the pressing concerns of AIDS in their own communities.

A concluding point of reflection: on the topic of international resources allotted for prevention, an intriguing development arose when one imam began speaking about funding from Islamic charities. Considering the activity of Islamic aid organizations, the imam noted that "They would come in for relief. They would fund maybe boreholes, water projects. They would fund expansion of a mosque or building mosques, and maybe *madrasas*. They are now funding a few educational institutions, quite a few. But issues of health has—for me—has not been a priority to them."[70] For this particular imam, the foreign resources for water projects and schools was donated in good faith, but in order to fully comprehend the needs of those Islamic leaders facing the crisis of HIV and AIDS in their own congregations, an open and more inclusive perspective is necessary, one that sees the epidemic in Nairobi as a priority.

In addressing the tension of accepting funds from foreign donors—both secular and Islamic—the issue becomes one of empowerment and being able to effectively meet the challenge of AIDS prevention in Nairobi. "Looking at the resources—I know the US government and the president's fund, the PEPFAR, has given a lot of money and I can assure you that the Muslims community has not received more than 1 percent of that—not even 1 percent of that has come to Kenya. Maybe because, of course, the ignorance on how to access the money within the community," noted the Muslim respondent on empowerment. "But I think there is the need to also just empower our communities that if there are resources, empower them on how to access those resources and utilize those resources effectively. So that has been our problem."[71]

To conclude this section, Muslim leaders in Nairobi see the need to empower not only their own communities, but they also need to empower themselves to be instruments of social change so that they can faithfully attend to the needs of the city's Muslim population. This empowerment involves strengthening the Islamic voice in prevention and reaching out to the Islamic aid organizations and charities to clarify the explicit needs for assistance, which can only be done from within the specific local setting and culture. For as this imam rightly illumines, what good is building a mosque if no one can attend services due to illness? Effective strategies are necessary for a comprehensive program on prevention to combat the AIDS crisis in Nairobi among the Muslim population. In establishing these objectives and working toward them collectively, the Muslims of Nairobi can mark the shift from crisis to *kairos*.

Prevention as *Kairos*

"I see the future being bright. But we still have to keep the tempo. There is a lot of good work going on. But if we slack behind there is the fear that the virus will erupt again. So, consistency has to be there," remarked one Muslim official working in advocacy. "We have to evaluate whatever we are doing so that—for the intention of keeping us on course. For the intention of identifying where the gaps are. For the intention of filling up the gaps we have. But I see lots of good things, the future is bright and we are better than what we were yesterday."[72] This optimistic assessment of efforts among the Islamic community in Nairobi highlights the movement from crisis to *kairos* historically. In terms of practical urgency, this sheikh self-consciously acknowledges that there is still work to be done—or "gaps" as he calls them.

In identifying that there are areas of activity that still need improvement, he offers a realistic picture of how religious leaders can practically come to terms with HIV in the Muslim community. This shift in perception on prevention efforts among Muslims can be seen in three major ways: by moving past a moralistic reading of the disease; by adapting ritual to allow for effective prevention among religious and medical workers; and by stressing the importance of Islamic officials in transforming how the general public sees HIV and people living with the virus.

From a historical perspective and similar to the trend in Catholicism, people who became infected initially kept quiet about their status, which in many ways led to a silent epidemic. Now, however, with imams and sheikhs talking about disease prevention, there have been some definite improvements in disease prevention. "Before ten years, before twenty years people used to hide themselves if they get that disease [HIV]. They did not want to be known," said one imam. "But nowadays, people go to their doctors, counselors."[73] One major conceptual shift during this period—from the early days of the epidemic in the mid- to late-1980s in Kenya—was a movement away from a moralistic view of how the disease was transmitted so that people living with infection can own their status and choose to live positively. In the words of another Islamic medical doctor representing the Muslim Health Secretariat, "As time goes and the epidemic—the pandemic really—there is realization that some very decent people who are not involved in anything are also getting infected. And therefore it is not just a matter of punishment for the wrongdoers, but the other people are getting infected and therefore we need to change our attitudes toward handling HIV. And that's where we are now."[74]

This change in view—that people who had not violated the moral principles of Islam were getting infected—is notable in that everyone, even sheikhs and imams, were susceptible to HIV and AIDS, and that there was no longer any one at-risk group in Nairobi, which then led to streamlined prevention efforts. The doctor continued, "[HIV] is something that we need to respond to in a different way. We need to prevent HIV from going on. We need to appreciate that HIV affects not only those wrongdoers, but also others who are innocent, whatever."[75] Again, addressing the underlying issues of morality and sexuality has enabled Muslim leaders to recognize that the epidemic is realistically a major problem for their community.

This acknowledgment comes in the face of erroneous view that the HIV prevalence rate was not as high in the Muslim community of Nairobi as in some other faith communities.[76] About this trend, the imam stated, "I think it is, you know Muslims—also looking backwards—they felt like this was not their people, so it was a problem of others."[77] Stressing the association between HIV infection and sexuality—a stigmatizing connection to be examined in the concluding chapter—many Muslim leaders early maintained that the disease was not an Islamic problem, that its spread was caused by a lack of virtue and morals, an acceptance of modernity, and cross-contamination of Islamic and Western values.[78] AIDS was thus considered a punishment for certain immoral actions and so faithful Muslims were immune to infection.

However, even in the view of this imam, there is the explicit affirmation that HIV infection is indeed a problem for the Muslim population of Nairobi when he said, "realizing the extent of the problem, and that Muslims are affected equally or maybe somehow maybe not as much as the others. But there is a realization that it is an issue that we need to understand better and to address and to participate also in addressing." He continued, "In the coastal area, where a lot of other people settled there because the local people are very accommodating even—and we have a kind of a cosmopolitan society. Then HIV also affects Muslims the same, maybe to a lesser degree, but in proportions that are equal to the proportion of the cosmopolitan societies."[79]

In a move to negotiate, construct, and maintain an Islamic identity in cosmopolitan Nairobi, Muslims are forced to confront the relationship between religious life and modernity. This involves the admission that HIV is a problem for Muslims—just as it is for Christians. The movement from prevention as crisis to prevention as *kairos* or opportunity, can be made with the understanding that HIV and AIDS are human problems and, with effective prevention models and methods, can be managed by Muslim leaders and health-care professionals. In one candid evaluation, the Muslim medical worker stated, "The situation now is while HIV is sort of no longer so much of an issue, people look at much more current diseases. Like on the coasts, there is dengue fever, there is whatever. But HIV has now become an ordinary citizen of the population of diseases. It's there, so it is there. Not so much concentration is given to HIV as such."[80] This citation, that HIV has "now become an ordinary citizen of the population of diseases," is remarkable in that this leader has genuinely accepted that HIV is a preventable, manageable, and treatable medical condition.

This belief that HIV is manageable also demonstrates a marked change in the way Muslim officials approach HIV infection, moving past the negative judgmental view of the disease to one that they can proactively prevent. Particularly in the field of health care, Islamic leaders are spearheading the discussion on ethics within their religious community, including such historically problematic issues as organ transplant and end of life care in relation to HIV and AIDS. "What Islam says is, life is not on your hands. You have to respect life. Therefore, give that patient painkillers to improve the quality of his life at that moment in time," said one sheikh. "But don't let him suffer with pain so that you can justify killing him. So there are issues—and it's case by case."[81] Reflecting on the practical nature of health care where difficult decisions must be made, he continued on to other areas of medical concern, "issues like transplant . . . like research, where you draw a line. Like you want to do research so that—like anything, HIV, ebola, whatever—so that you can help generations to come. So, how do you go about it?"[82]

He concluded, "organ transplant, like a kidney—since you can still live with one kidney, and provide life to another person whose life is in danger—

they [Muslim jurists] say 'That is something which is supposed to be done.' "[83] In respecting life, this Islamic educator offered a very liberal view of organ donation and transplant, one that is not necessarily agreed upon throughout the Muslim world. And yet he echoes the preceding comments, that HIV is by nature no different than any other chronic condition—particularly not from a moral standpoint—and the work being done now by Muslims in the field of health care and prevention will in reality aid future generations yet to come.

In an interdisciplinary effort, Muslim imams and doctors are working together to implement measures to prevent disease transmission both in the mosque and in the hospital. For example, the use of white, latex gloves in ritual ceremonies which was once considered to be an explicit affirmation that the person was HIV positive is now commonplace for both childbirth and in Muslim funeral ceremonies (Arabic, *janazah*). Given the broad range of childbearing techniques informed by culture, religion, and ethnicity—some women opt to go to the hospital while others choose to consult a midwife and have the birth at home—there have been some distinct changes in preventative practices. According to one Islamic health-care worker, there has been an increase in "the small precautionary measures in the handling of childbirth, for example,. Even when it is handled traditionally they use gloves and things like that are common practices now, even among the traditional methods of traditional birth attendance and so on. There is marked concern for hygienic practices, for protection from infection, so on."[84]

This change in medical procedure, long since adopted by hospitals and medical workers, now signals a trend in adopting precautionary methods to prevent HIV and AIDS infection. From both a Western and traditional medicine vantage point, there is distinct headway being made, especially in Islamic health care. A similar shift in focus is occurring in the mosques where imams are familiarizing themselves with the physiological dimensions of HIV and AIDS infection and are adopting practices to forestall transmission. This imam who officiates over the Islamic preparation of the body for burial asserted, "People are now more conscious on handling the dead and so on. And I think equipment have been put in place in mosques, because handling the dead is a mosque affair in every community so you find gloves and things like that. And the use of disinfectant which were not previously used are now commonplace."[85]

In an interesting sociological development, the use of latex gloves simply and powerfully marks the shift in HIV and AIDS prevention from crisis to *kairos*. For, while these gloves were once historically associated with moralistic judgment, their usage now is widely accepted as an effective precaution against infection. And where procedures and rituals marking birth and death are intimate events that deeply affect the identity of the Muslims, this religious community in Nairobi as a whole recognizes the possible threat of HIV and AIDS infection and has methodologically moved to decrease the likelihood of contracting the disease in the course of performing their professional responsibilities.

Islamic leaders—doctors, midwives, imams, and sheikhs—are thus instrumental in instituting change within the Muslim population of Nairobi regarding which prevention initiatives are effective and areas that might need to be developed further. In terms of actual influence, however, the imams of Kenya hold tremendous sway over how their congregations perceive the epidemic and some have even gone so far as to speak about HIV from the *minbar*, or the pulpit found in the mosque. Yet this was not always a welcome message from religious officials. Remarking on the historical change in how HIV infection was viewed in the mosque, the representative from the Muslim Health Secretariat noted, "I will answer that question [on the HIV and AIDS prevention efforts from within Islam] in historical perspective. In the early stages of this epidemic, a Muslim imam may lose credibility with his audience or congregation if he spoke to his congregation so often on HIV."[86]

This is a tragic historical consequence since it was during the early days of the epidemic when the most amount of information and advocacy would have been most effective. Yet, losing credibility would cause the congregation to question the legitimacy of the imam in leading the mosque. Truly, then, this was a crisis of prevention. "But this has since changed," affirmed the imam. "One of my roles also is to educate the imams to be able to communicate the challenges to those who are not very well-informed in the health aspect [of the epidemic]. So a lot has been done to train the imams so that they can be confident enough to talk to their congregation about HIV and any other diseases as such."[87]

Kenyan imams are singularly influential in espousing and shaping the views of the religious community, since, as we have already seen, "people put their trust in their religious leaders more than ever—some trust them even more than they trust their own parents."[88] Because of the influence that they hold over popular opinion, one other interesting shift in scope has been the imamate recommending that Muslim couples who are to be married go to the hospital and get tested. On the topic of VCT, an imam employed at one of the largest mosques in Nairobi saw that, for Muslim engaged couples, testing for HIV infection should be a prerequisite, even if to "just know their status so that, whatever the outcome, they know what they are getting into. And they can be guided."[89] As a religious leader, the imam can guide and teach couples how to prevent future infection by knowing their status.

In yet another proactive measure, this imam recollects working with other Islamic officials, "We had a forum of the registrars, the *kadis*, registrars of marriages, we were talking about—then insisting that before maybe we issue the marriage certificate which is an important document, you should prove to us that you've actually undergone HIV and AIDS test." He continued regarding the obstacles in adopting and preaching such an approach to HIV prevention, "It is very difficult to enforce it, because of the laws, they—you cannot discriminate against somebody. So you cannot force somebody, you can only guide them and advise them. We were telling the imams to use the pulpit, or the *minbar*, to talk about it and just sensitize people."[90]

For this imam engaged in advocacy—both within the mosque and within the broader community—prevention is a strategic objective since the health of the individual affects the overall health of the Muslim community in Nairobi. However, the strength of the message for prevention as *kairos* is only as strong as the imam's understanding of HIV infection. The imam goes further, saying:

> We have several interventions going on within the community and these people are going around and guiding people on the need to check their status and also they need not to stigmatize those who have been affected. Because no more. You cannot judge, you cannot tell people how they are affected and why. So all we do is together is to receive them. So the imam has that role. Because if one of the parents dies, they will rush to the imam for support—to look for support, for the orphans who are left behind. So it all comes back to the imam and therefore there is of course the need for the imam to really understand, and how to respond to these issues, and how to ensure that they guide the community to minimize the rate of infection. Because that will, again, minimize the challenges that come to them.[91]

Minimizing challenges thus represents one of the more difficult conceptual challenges for these Muslim leaders, one that again considers the negotiation and construction of Islamic identity in modern Nairobi.

Of course with the discussion of modernity, Muslim leaders must consider the place of Muslim youth in such an urban setting. That is, how do imams attempt to reinforce orthodox Islamic belief, teaching, and practice about HIV and AIDS infection in a location of social and ideological flux such as Nairobi? "As we say, prevention is better than cure. First of all, we sensitize our Muslim communities, especially youth, to abstain. Because prevention is better than cure. You know, the majority of youth have been affected especially in colleges already positive there. So we sensitize them to prevent until they get married, so they're going to do sex—then they have to get married first of all," said one imam working for the Kenyan Council of Imams. "After that, other prevention—because our religion, especially I think you know about Islam—our Prophet Muhammad, *ṣalla llāhu ʿalayhi wa-alehe wa-sallam,* urged Muslim youth to get married. If you are not able, what they do they fast. You get fasting—you know fasting? Yeah they fast because the fasting will prevent them [from premarital sex]."[92]

With this statement, the imam reinforces Islamic values regarding popular attitudes involving premarital sex and marriage and the ritual prescription of fasting to prevent illicit sexual activity. And yet, even with this standard of behavior—that all youth will eschew the temptation of sexual relations and the modernity of college—other imams see that there is a practical dimension in the *kairos* of prevention—that even if someone is infected, they are not condemned according to Islamic teaching. Through collaboration between Muslim doctors and religious leaders, the Muslim population in Nairobi can collectively respond to HIV infection and actually engage in prevention efforts together. "So especially, a Muslim doctor—they do counseling," noted the imam. "Maybe somebody came with that problem, HIV/AIDS. So it will not spread because they are here."[93]

The tone of this comment demonstrates that AIDS is an issue in the Muslim community and that through effective prevention efforts it can be adequately addressed and mitigated. As for the Muslim youth who are daily confronted with the challenge of constructing an Islamic identity in a city setting, this imam advocates for VCT so that the couple can know their statues before getting married. In a move toward transparency, he advised, "to tell our youth before they get married, we maybe call them for counseling and we solicit them to go for a test before they get married."[94] This view, that Muslim couples who wish to be wed should get tested represents the theological advancement from the crisis of the early days of the AIDS epidemic when those living with infection were met with judgment, denial, and silence from the Islamic leadership. Now, even for those who fear they might be HIV positive, the imam championed that, "because we feared that somebody would be infected, then they say, 'Not me, you will bring me there [to the VCT center].' Before we get married, we call them if they accept. And then we tell them, 'Go for counseling.' Because we make the provision for that."[95]

The influence and authority of the imams in Nairobi has been instrumental in how the Muslim population has understood and continues to understand AIDS prevention strategies, even in the face of fear. In this way, the imamate promotes the communal life of the *'ummah* (Arabic for the Muslim community) by giving people the resources, the vocabulary, and the support to deal with HIV and AIDS in their daily lives—most notably here in the opportunity of disease prevention.

To conclude this section, one imam working in the area of HIV and AIDS prevention in Nairobi, offers this critical insight on the crossroads between theology and medicine:

> In Islam, we respond to it as the way we respond to any other disease. If you have been infected by HIV, you are advised to go and go to doctor or whatever, and he will guide you on how to take care of your body, or how to hygienic

> issues. What to eat, what not to eat. Like any other disease, you don't just say that because you are a Muslim now you don't have to go to hospital. We even encourage people to use these ARV's to keep themselves fit. So we don't only rely on spiritual whatever. But we have also to work hard with the doctors to make sure that the guy is fit well.[96]

The above quotation insinuated that the era of HIV exceptionalism is over, thanks in large part to those Islamic leaders working in health care and prevention. And, as the imam notes, this involves an interdisciplinary method, one that involves both Muslim official leadership and Muslim medical professionals. Islamic prevention efforts—moving away from morally judging people with HIV and AIDS, a change in ritual and understanding of the disease, and positively employing the office of the imam in changing people's views about the epidemic—has shifted focus from darkness to light, from crisis to *kairos*.

Education as Crisis

"It depends on the perception. If you perceive HIV to be a punishment from Allah, then someone will view it as a justice. Then—you think of the child. The innocent kid who was born with HIV and AIDS. For that case, would you categorize it as being justice for the kid? That's a question for me myself."[97] This self-conscious reflection from one Muslim respondent fundamentally addresses the crisis in HIV and AIDS education. That is, the crisis involves how the Islamic leadership has been able to address and change common misconceptions and moralistic judgments toward those Kenyans living with infection in the sphere of education, particularly when the disease involves theological notions such as divine justice and punishment.

In terms of education, one of the most pressing concerns lies in disseminating factual information about HIV and AIDS, and how every population—both Islamic and otherwise—is susceptible to infection. For one Islamic leader in Nairobi, the challenge lies in being able to see and differentiate between fact and misinformation as it relates to the HIV and AIDS education program within the Muslim community. "First and foremost, the response is to give the right information so that you remove the misconception about HIV," the subject stated. "You want to give the factual information, because up until now I think—and this is my personal opinion—that the communities, or the people on the ground, they don't have factual information."[98]

Because people have not been taught about the disease in a credible manner, this imam sees that one major obstacle lies in educating the population scientifically correct information about modes of disease transmission. Addressing the relationship between Islam and modernity, he noted that people might think they know about HIV and AIDS risk in a very general sense. "They might have information, because they heard it on the radio, they've seen it on TV. But it's just very general information. When you go to the quality of that information, to the detail—there is a lot of gray areas," he said. "So it is the responsibility of religious leaders, whether they are imams, pastors, or priests, or fathers, or bishops, or whatever—first and foremost, for them to be educated, get the right information. Level two, to pass that information to their congregations. I think it's very, very important."[99]

This observation points once again to the fact that there are many different modes of education—from the secular governmental that incorporates mass media into its strategy, to the religious that tries to make sense of the disease in a spiritual way and which, in some ways, may lead to an apparent disparity between general and specific knowledge about the disease. This creates a rather difficult landscape to navigate, where the Muslim population of Nairobi is familiar with general facts about risk but not knowledgeable on the specific information on HIV infection and transmission.

This same imam goes on to identity the conceptual dichotomy between education efforts in the countryside and in Nairobi, when he said, "I believe the small villages are manageable. Information spreads fast. If you yourself go to a small village, within a half an hour everybody will know *mzungu* [KiSwahili for 'white person'] has come. So small villages they are manageable." However, "big cities like Nairobi, it's very hard you see to manage. You have people with different ideas, not necessarily respecting the religious leader's view. Not necessarily. So I think it's a bit different from other places."[100] This distinction between country and city life, is important in the discussion on the crisis of education since it identifies the limitations of educational scope and setting.

That is, in smaller villages, it is logistically much easier to collectively teach a unified message about HIV to the population. In Nairobi, however, it is significantly more difficult to keep on message with a population of over three million. Consequently, urban life has its own challenges in the area of HIV and AIDS education from an Islamic perspective. And yet even in Kenya's capital city, where educational initiatives would seem to be more effective given the broad depth of secular and religious influences and resources, there remain certain indigenous African understandings of the disease—such as it being a curse or punishment for the violation of social order. In the estimation of one sheikh originally from Kisii in Western Kenya, there exists a spectrum of education and authority in Nairobi among the leadership which affects how the disease is understood in the various communities.

"Of course there is a difference between those who are learned and those who are not learned. For the learned person, his understanding of HIV will be better than the usual person in the street. The same thing applies in Islam," said the sheikh. "There are those who are much learned, they know more about HIV than those who are just there. When it is time for you to make them understand what Islam says about HIV, some of them believe maybe it is a curse and it has no cure and you don't have to discuss it. And they don't know fact from knowledge."[101] That the disease is still considered to be the result of some curse or punishment demonstrates a lack of evidential knowledge on disease etiology. Even with the foundational Islamic teachings that forbid religious practice outside of orthodoxy, some imams and sheikhs acknowledge that culture and traditional views on HIV hinder many educational methods.

Speaking on these trends examined in the first part of this chapter—namely witchcraft, sorcery, and ancestor worship—one imam considered these practices as "*haram* [Arabic for 'forbidden'] but it happens. Even here in Nairobi, not only in rural areas—even in Nairobi, even though they are against Islam's teachings."[102] Here the subject makes the conceptual distinction between life in the rural areas and life in the city, as well as how these two identities can prove problematic in educating the Muslim population about the virus. Another imam echoed this sentiment, looking at the indigenous elements at work in how people come to terms with HIV, saying, "Maybe because people where they grew up, they grew up in a village whereby this traditional medicine man also is still operating. So these kind of beliefs—although he might be a Muslim or a Christian, but those beliefs, also they are still in the background. So, maybe it has an effect. But generally, when somebody is desperate, then anything you tell him, he will believe, he will say, 'That's true.' "[103]

This account sheds some light on why people would venture outside of mainstream Islamic teaching in an attempt to find a remedy for HIV. Since there is no known cure for the disease, instead of giving way to despair those infected search for a reason to keep their hope alive in the form of indigenous belief. And this is where Islamic education may prove beneficial in combatting some of the negative stereotypes regarding the epidemic to provide factual information for the Muslim population of Nairobi. "Now, there is a lot of information. Of course, these things always occur when they don't have factual information. But as we are getting more informed and more informed, then people—they kind of shy away from these [traditional] practices," the imam continued. "Because even in the medical sector, I think, people didn't have a lot of information. So they themselves also feared to handle a dead body. They will—everybody will fear to handle that dead body because they fear to be infected. But as people are more educated and more educated these things are being shunned away."[104]

Regarding the historical dimension of the crisis of HIV and AIDS education at an early stage, even those working in the field of medicine and health care did not have suitable education on the risks of HIV and AIDS. This lack of information in the early days of the epidemic represents one of the myriad elements leading to the failure of Islamic leaders to come to the aid of those infected, instead espousing and citing miseducation as fact. But, as the imam acknowledged, some of this misinformation is being addressed by Muslim leaders who are teaching their congregations about effective prevention about HIV transmission.

These educational efforts, in many cases, are geared toward changing some of the attitudes and ideas that ethnic and cultural communities have about HIV and AIDS. In this way, education is necessary to inform religious practice, particularly in Islam. "[Traditional worship] is there. It's less though because there's a great punishment. We are told that one of the greatest sins that God will not forgive is being associated with a partner . . . *shirk*. So if you go to a *mganga*, then you are associating God with a partner. But it is there, we can't deny it in the rural areas and—let me tell you—even in the urban areas," said one leader identifying the basic dilemma of rectifying traditional worship with Islam. "There are people who don't believe they can live without having consulted the *mganga*, the traditional *mganga*, to tell them about their life, wealth, and all that. So it is there. We cannot deny it. "Although the sheikhs are doing their best to tell them, 'You cannot rely on anybody else apart from God,' because the person you are going to is also a creation of God."[105]

Through consulting a traditional healer, for some scholars, is an Islamic sin, it adds an interesting sociological dimension to the crisis of HIV and AIDS in Kenya since, in many ways, it influences how many Kenyans identify themselves religiously. Clearly, it is a challenge for Muslims leaders in that under the Islamic belief in the principle of *tawhīd*, going to the *mganga* is not a part of official, sanctioned Islamic practice. In the same way as faith healers who lay hands on people living with HIV infection give healing, many of these traditional healers offer their services for some fee and promise to cure them of disease. These diviners are dealing with a grim exchange of goods—money for hope—but there is, to date, no known cure for HIV and AIDS, only treatments. Islamic educators are thus faced with the crisis of teaching the population that the *mganga* cannot cure the disease and they should instead consult their qualified medical officials for an effective drug regimen.

One element of this crisis involves ignorance of the severity of the epidemic, or the belief that one is not susceptible to infection. The imam concluded, "I think it is—in terms of perception, 'we' cannot get it. I think it's there. But its more to do with ignorance. I'll tell you among, for example, the Somali community. They couldn't believe that somebody can have HIV/AIDS."[106] Marking the distinction between culture, ethnicity, and religion, this Muslim leader makes that point that certain groups view the risk of contracting the disease differently—in this case Somalis which represent not only an external nationality but also a different ethnicity even though the majority of the Somali population is Muslim—once again emphasizing the crisis of AIDS education.

Regarding Islamic teaching on HIV, one central challenge concerns the question of how Muslim educators can change the view that certain groups believe themselves to be incapable of contracting the disease—whether influenced by culture, religion, or ethnicity. This belief, certainly not specific to the Somali community living in Nairobi, is reinforced by other Muslim leaders who cite certain ethnic rites and rituals that lead to an increased potential of infection. While much has been written on the practice of levirate marriage in the Luo ethnic group,[107] one imam working in HIV prevention sees a connection between culture and ethnicity. "There are certain cultures, for example, in the Luo—the Luo culture. Because of their ethnicity, they also have certain cultures. Therefore their culture, for example,—allows for wife inheritance. So, in that perspective, irrespective of what the husband died of, that widow is inherited by the next brother," affirmed the imam. "And that widow might be HIV positive, and the Luo don't want to know. They will inherit, and in the process they will have sexual contact and this will infect others."[108] This Luo practice, while denounced by both Islamic leaders, government officials, and medical professionals, still continues.

Though an analysis of this practice on gender roles and sexual expectations is out of the scope of this section, another Islamic leader working in education marks the distinction between Islam as a religion and the cultural practices performed by people who profess to be Muslim, saying "there are issues that are cultural but are not Islamic. For example, female circumcision. It's not Islamic, but those who do it are Muslims. So there is sometimes an overlap and there is sometimes a conflict also between culture and traditions and Islamic faith."[109] This acknowledgment that there is no one clear sense of being Muslim is a useful reminder when looking at the challenge of education on HIV and AIDS in Nairobi. Hence, education has been problematized in terms of misinformation about the disease, the popular perception of modern life in Nairobi, and now even in terms of culture.

There exists a gradient scale of those Muslims who follow the religious laws of Islam, those that practice female genital mutilation (FGM), those that are Somali, those that consult the *mganga*, and in reality countless other variations and aberrations of Islamic practice in Kenya's capital city. Regarding levirate marriage and Islamic conceptions, the subject continued, "some tribes are more conservative than others in their sexual behaviors and practices. While Islam consolidates the practices and behaviors, where you have strong cultural influence the Muslims also are affected. For example, in Nyanza [the county located in the southwest corner of Kenya], they have wife inheritance, they have whatever. So this also affects how people see Muslims throughout the region."[110] Marking the difference between religion and culture may prove useful in education efforts since separating the two might make it easier to identify the Islamic teaching needed to positively affect belief and practice aimed at preventing future infection.

As the imam rightly states, learned Islam prescribes a certain course of action particularly when it comes to sexuality. Yet, given the practical example of wife inheritance in Nyanza—a practice that is by its very nature, culturally and ethnically conditioned—the Muslim population living in this geographic location or coming from this ethnic group may find it difficult to reconcile religion and culture. Education, then, can serve as a helpful tool for addressing questions of both a religious, ethnic, and cultural nature. The locus of these efforts within the Muslim community in Nairobi rests on Islamic educators and leaders to lead the charge in dispelling misinformation and cultural conceptions of HIV and AIDS.

Whereas education is an iterative process—influenced by complex factors such as culture, curricula, ideology, prevailing notions, and myriad other elements—one of the most important influences in the process is the actual educator. And, within Islam, the educators and the educational process are inherently tied to religious leadership. "I think it is the issue of leadership. The current leadership we have, I think, is not very strong. Initially, religious leaders would play their role as people who are there to guide the community," said one sheikh involved in curriculum development for national Islamic Religious Education (IRE). "But now, religious leaders are taking political sides. So either a politician is from your community, then you don't talk about the ills he's committing. So, very fast the religious leadership is losing that moral authority. And the adherents have nobody to turn to."[111]

This sheikh sees the conflation of religion and politics as particularly problematic in terms of claiming moral authority which negatively affects how religious figures are perceived by the community. This thereby jeopardizes their influence in the field of education. "What I think should happen is that religious leadership now should come up and be strong and be firm. And define their role very prominently, in terms of—if you are speaking against justice or injustice, we have to speak against injustice," he continued. "It doesn't matter where the injustice affects, or who it affects. We have to have certain standards where we all live by."[112] Such an ecumenical statement serves to address the major challenge of education as it offers the chance of hope for Islamic leaders and educators to actively influence not only what is being taught, but also how it is being taught—particularly as this relates to HIV and AIDS prevention in Kenya. This shift in focus for Islamic education, from challenge to opportunity, is precisely what this chapter now examines in the next section, education as *kairos*.

Education as *Kairos*

"The good news is that we have integrated, we just talk freely about it [HIV and AIDS] nowadays. As in, when the issue of HIV comes—these are everyday issues. . . . But nowadays you don't even have to have a specific lecture or sermon on that. It comes in different issues, it is just integrated," asserted one Muslim educator representing the Kenyan Council of Imams.[113] This observation identifies the conceptual shift among the Muslims of Nairobi, away from the era of AIDS exceptionalism to an integrated approach where the disease is understood in daily terms which informs how religious educators teach about the disease in the classroom.

Clearly, one of the most important elements of education as *kairos*—or as an opportunity for change—involves what exactly is being taught and by whom. Reflected one imam:

> In the *madrasa*, they should teach everything. And for me I believe strong religion—if people understand their values, their religious values—then many of the challenges we have today would be addressed. Challenges of poverty. Challenges of disease. We cannot say, "You'll not contract HIV and AIDS just because you believe, because you have strong moral values or religious values." Because it could be true, you could contract [HIV] on accident, whatever. But we are saying that maybe understanding can lessen some of those challenges. So [the imams] should understand how you get it. What I know is that there was a time I did a program with the *madrasa* teachers on HIV and AIDS and we did ask them that they could mention some of those things within the *madrasas* that could help explain transmission. The only challenge is that we don't have many who were empowered enough to go out and do that. But we have exposed quite a number to training.[114]

Even from an institutional level, the way that HIV and AIDS is being treated academically overlaps to a large degree with religious teachings. The influence of Islamic leaders, then, is of tremendous significance on the content of what is being taught in the *madrasa* since it serves both as a religious establishment and an educational facility. For this reason, the sheikh serves a dual purpose as leader of both religion and education.

On the legitimacy that Kenyans ascribe to their religious leaders, one imam working in curriculum development in IRE, noted on the dichotomy of politics and religion, "even politicians, people—they don't trust them so much. Although they are also part of the leadership—it's the political leadership. But religious leaders are held into esteem, therefore whatever they say it has some weight."[115] Having spoken to many imams engaged in educational efforts throughout Nairobi, there was a consensus that they should use their position of authority to teach the Muslim population about HIV and AIDS.

One sheikh spoke particularly of his experience working with other Islamic leaders financed by the Global Fund through Care International. The strategy they adopted in the mosque, "was to use the religious leaders to reach out to the community. They somehow created awareness, so they used to talk about it—sensitization, trainings. There are some cases whereby we involved them to be facilitators for the trainings."[116] This marks a critical development in AIDS education for the Muslim population of Nairobi, since it allowed these religious leaders to address the epidemic on their own terms by actually admitting that HIV is a problem for their community of faithful. This then empowers the Islamic officials to be agents of social change in their local communities, signaling the theological dimensions of *kairos*. "For the imam and the sheikh, their role is to handle the issues of HIV on a religious perspective. And how to impress each other in case maybe one of the family member of the community is affected," affirmed this sheikh involved in the education process. "Their role is to give out the religious perspective concerning how to take care of the sick, and the—in short how to fight the stigma. They play a crucial role of encouraging people to be together."[117]

Remarking on the significance of religious leadership in community-building and how the disease is internalized by the Muslim population, this sheikh sees that the religious leadership—the sheikhs and imams—have an integral part to play in education and even helping to ease the sting of stigma. In any case, Muslim officials in Nairobi occupy a very influential position in relation to HIV and AIDS education. To reinforce his sentiment on the integrated approach necessary to positively teach people about risk and transmission, the sheikh concluded, "The teaching for the community is associated with the religious teaching. It's in one way or another, they are intertwined."[118] In this way, the grassroots approach to education initiatives are inherently tied to religious education and, according to this Islamic official, both are interrelated.

Similarly, this belief underscores the interdisciplinary nature of the lived religious response of Muslim leadership toward the AIDS epidemic in that neither secular nor religious education is mutually exclusive. Rather, each discipline is informed by the other resulting in a hybrid mix of cultural, ethnic, social, and indeed religious elements. Because of this, education in Nairobi is at a crossroads and those Muslim leaders confronting the epidemic in their daily lives are instrumental in disseminating factually correct information about the disease to their congregations. "Religious leaders have an impact—positive impact—toward the community in terms of persistence, reminder. I'll say a reminder. Because if you are being reminded about being faithful, for example, to your one partner. And then fearing Allah," in the prescient yet candid words of this sheikh on the movement in the field of education from crisis to *kairos*. "It would be an impact to the community. And then the spread—the spread of HIV at least would be confined. Then, on the negative side, if I told the religious leaders that I've not been able to undergo training and understand the issue of HIV and AIDS." He continued, "If they are stigmatized, self-stigma, then their impact is negative to the community. So it's a two-way, either positive through persistence, reminder. Then the negative, they discriminate."[119]

In this insightful analysis, the sheikh highlights the integrated nature of Islamic teaching on HIV since there is not much difference between the community and the Islamic perspective regarding the epidemic and, often, the Muslim community is guided by Islamic leaders who are in turn influenced by Islamic teachings. Yet, as the sheikh rightly notes, this can have both a positive and a negative impact for the Muslim community in viewing educational efforts as either a crisis or an opportunity. The Islamic leaders and educators are thus integral figures in this process of education.

In practice, Muslim officials are also influential since they are not only the ones who speak to people about various aspects of the disease—risk, transmission, stigma, VCT—but they also relate to the Muslim population on a daily basis, in human terms, since they often know these people living within the community as neighbors. Said one imam on the influence of Islamic educators, "Actually we have had quite a number of congregational talks on HIV and AIDS. We've had programs which target specifically imams and just to empower them on how to talk and handle issues of HIV and AIDS." Regarding the intimate knowledge and fiduciary relationship that the imam or sheikh maintains with the Islamic community in Nairobi, he continued, "The imams of course have received these issues on a daily basis because they are the ones who preside over burials, they are the ones who preside over marriages. And therefore we are also telling them, before they preside over marriage, they should advise the couples to have an HIV test."[120]

Naturally, educational initiatives aimed at sensitizing imams and sheikhs are critical in the overall Islamic strategy for providing care for the whole human person. And, as these leaders are interacting with the Muslim population of Nairobi in their daily lives—even officiating over the most important events in a person's life, ceremonies marking birth, marriage, and death—they are seen as credible voices in the discourse surrounding AIDS education. It is through bringing their views on HIV infection in accordance with medically accurate diagnoses of the disease that these figures in the field of Islamic education and empowerment can change popular notions of disease risk and transmission, thereby moving past moralistic judgments on those Muslims living with the virus.

Reflecting on the practical response to HIV and AIDS in the Muslim population of Kenya's capital, religious leaders have gone so far as to discuss the issues of education during the Friday *jum`ah* prayer in many of the large mosques in Nairobi. In one mosque located in downtown Nairobi where men aspiring to be imams attend seminary training to obtain a *ijazah* certificate to lead their own congregations, mosque officials offer seminars on HIV and AIDS education—how it is acquired, how it is treated—so that when these imams return to their mosque they can teach about the epidemic from an educated vantage point. "For example, imams are being called here for seminaries—to teach them about HIV. How you can acquire HIV, programs to understand," asserted one imam on this development in education. "But when you go back to the local mosque, the same information you are given here are the ones that you are going to preach there. So we have seminars on HIV. Even some of the imams have gone as far as discussing it through media—radio programs, and quite frankly, TV programs."[121]

The cumulative effect of this opportunity for transformative education among the Muslim population of Nairobi is exponential since teaching one sheikh or one imam the medical dimensions about the virus has the potential of changing the opinions of innumerable others. The onus of this formulation, thus, lays in large part on the local imam and sheikh to seek out these educational seminars on sensitization and empowerment to address the issue of AIDS in their own congregations with some expertise.[122] Expressed differently by another Muslim official regarding the privileged yet unique relationship between the imam and the congregation, "I might preach in the mosque. I tell you this and this. So it is upon you to go and implement what you've learned in the mosque in your house. I can't come in your house and tell your wife and kids. So, if there's no good operation between the congregation and the imams, of course we will fail in our work."[123]

This is a rather compelling observation, that even if the imam preaches about HIV and AIDS to his congregation, the real work remains to be done by the constituent members of the community. In this way, the community by its nature is made up of individual persons, which the imam identifies when he followed, "What we need is good connection between the imams and the congregation and also, you as an individual. You start from your personal level, you see? You make sure that your kids are living a good way, you teach them good behaviors. Because I can't come in your house and do everything for you," he concluded. "So it is a challenge, you speak in the mosque but the implementation on the ground—that's what we expect from the people."[124] Changing the hearts and the minds of the individual Muslim to act according to the message of Islam—through works of mercy, hospitality, and justice—is a major challenge for the transformative power of education.

Though central to any real educational efforts, the instruction is only as legitimate and effective as its source. For Islam specifically, the strength of the educational message and method based in Islamic scripture—the Qur'ān, *Hadith*, and *Sunnah*—provide some of the strongest justifications for Muslim belief in the purpose of sickness and epidemic. These sources also provide the grounds for religious officials to justify and legitimate their views regarding HIV and AIDS. When applied to the epidemic in Kenya, the result is a predominately positive scriptural analysis that affirms the inherent dignity of the individual living with infection.

From this, there are three major areas of Islamic teaching that mark the movement from crisis to *kairos*: the injunction to visit the sick; viewing disease as a test from God; and the Islamic belief that every disease has a cure which may or may not yet be known to humanity. In general for Islam, in the words of one interlocutor, “There are teachings that prohibit discrimination. There are teachings that we need to take care of our sick, irrespective of whatever. There are teachings on being merciful to others.”[125] These teachings based in the Qur’ān and *Hadith* traditions have their own legitimacy regarding how the Muslim population of Nairobi should view and treat people living with the disease. From the interviews, the sheikhs and imams used positive scriptural support related to disease in the foundational sources of Islamic theology to correct negative views of the disease as well as their views regarding people living with the disease.

For example, according to one imam, one of the quintessential *Hadith* used by Islamic leaders attending to the sick in their congregations reads, “one of the teachings says that on the Day of Judgment, Allah will ask you ‘I was sick and you did not visit me.’ Then he will ask, ‘Allah, how could you have been sick?’ He will say, ‘One of my creations was sick and you didn’t visit them.’ And therefore there is a lot, actually we have right now *sheikhs* who go around to hospitals just praying for people.” The imam concluded, “There is a lot of reward for Muslims to visit the sick and take care of the sick.”[126] Just as this *Hadith* makes clear and the imam explicitly references, there is the widespread belief that visiting the sick of this world will benefit you in the next.

Indicating the theological link between positive scripture and those imams and sheikhs charged with teaching people how to understand the Islamic notions of disease, the imam cited the *Hadith* tradition of the Prophet Muhammad, “There are quite a number [of *Hadith* traditions] in terms of visiting the sick, taking care of the sick. And the reward you get from it.”[127] This correlation based in the Islamic leader’s own theology is crucial in understanding the importance of both the medical professional and the Islamic educator in treating the human person, which also points to the interdisciplinary and interdependent strategy adapted in the *kairos* of Islamic education in Nairobi.

Stemming from this interpretation, the subject brought up another *Hadith* which reads, “of course, God says He created every disease with a cure. So we also say that one of these days, we will find the cure. Because God does not lie—He tells us that there is a cure for every disease, if only people knew. So maybe we have not reached that level, but with scientists we will soon be there.”[128] It may be obvious at this point that—as a transition from darkness to light, from crisis to *kairos*—the AIDS epidemic in Kenya is not an issue that can be fully treated solely in terms of theology or medicine. Rather, as the *Hadith* exactly asserts, it is the work of doctors and religious leaders to come together—motivated by the grace and almighty power of God—to discover the social, spiritual, and physiological medical remedies for those living with disease.

Accordingly, another sheikh also references this *Hadith*, this time directly related to HIV and AIDS when he said, "Of course the Messenger of Islam has told us that, HIV—and every disease—has a cure. And we believe in it because it is an adoration from Allah. So we believe *In shā' Allāh* here is a cure for it and Allah's Messengers do not say anything that is far away from fact. They say fact all the time."[129] This tradition offers legitimacy to the claim that God has appointed a cure to every disease since this *Hadith* is attributed to the Prophet Muhammad and encourages Islamic religious leaders in teaching positively about the epidemic in Nairobi.

However, it is true that scripture can be used to justify many different theological beliefs. Take, for example, the view that disease is a punishment from God:

> Of course scripture there, we believe that HIV/ADS—ok we as Muslims, we can say that HIV/AIDS, we can put it into two perspectives. First, it just a disease. That it can get you. Second, we can say maybe because there is veneration of Allah that says, "When people start doing sins openly, and announcing it aloud, we punish them with a disease that was not there, for the people who were there before them." So we can say, first it is just a disease. You can be tested just like other disease. Second, we can say it is a punishment from Allah because of our own sins. So we have scriptures from the Qur'ān to use, we have scriptures from the *Hadith* to use to discuss the matters.[130]

This imam makes a binary distinction on the nature of disease—as a treatable medical condition or as a punishment from God. To overlook that such a view of illness exists would be irresponsible from that theological perspective.[131] Nevertheless, one other respondent, a prominent religious figure in Nairobi, simply responded in opposition to this view, "there were people believing that the disease was a punishment from Allah. But now that has changed."[132] This view marks a shift in the perception of AIDS within the Muslim population in Nairobi, from the disease as a punishment from God to one that may be best described as a test, requiring patience on the part of those negatively affected by the epidemic.

"We also know that whatever situation befalls one actually you are told that if you fall sick sometimes it's good for you because God is washing away your sins. So that could also be a way. And therefore don't look at people falling sick, especially from HIV and AIDS as people who are already condemned—that they have another opportunity to use that time to repent and do nice things," attested one other Muslim interlocutor. "We have quite a number of scriptures that talk about disease and talk about people not judging people. Of course, and also a number of teaching in terms of from the Prophet."[133] This response runs the theological gamut for the *kairos* of effective theological education based in Islamic scripture—dispensation for sins, movement away from condemnation, repentance. In this articulation, the actual human person is being confronted by the very real challenges of life on earth, which, in essence, is a realistic analysis of the experience of those living with infection.

While it still carries some weight of moral judgment in Islamic terms, this subject presents the view in positive terms, that sins will be washed away if the Muslim faithful performs "nice things." Reflecting on the spiritual notion of human agency, the lesson some Islamic leaders propose for those living with infection is to develop the spiritual virtue of patience. On the topic of AIDS education as representing a movement from crisis to *kairos*—or from despair to hope—the Islamic leader involved in educational efforts within the *madrasas* in Nairobi offered this consideration:

> If you feel as a human person, something is not good, then have patience. And God tells us, "Whatever befalls you, say 'thank you.' And from God we came, to Him we will return." You know, you don't go moaning. So, it is a favor that has befallen us. That's, for me, how I would look at it. The human in me might say, "Well, how can I . . . ? How can it be . . . ?" But if you look at it from that spiritual perspective, you look at it as a favor. And therefore it's either going to take you to paradise or hellfire, the way you handle it. Do you disbelieve in God now? Do you start going to *mganga*? Or do you tell God to give you more patience, or to give you to lessen the pain and the burden? You know, and just thank Him for that situation. So me, that's how I take it.[134]

This belief, past judgment to a realistic understanding of the human condition, demonstrates a change in the way the Muslim community perceives AIDS, due in large part to empowered and sensitized imams such as this one. Accordingly, one of the central elements of the *kairos* of education lies in destigmatization efforts. Or, in the words of another Islamic respondent, "Things are changing now. Ten years ago, things were different. Now things have changed."[135] The next, third and final section, will consider the historical crisis and contemporary *kairos* of destigmatization efforts within the Islamic leadership in Nairobi.

Destigmatization as Crisis

"Of course such cases are there, where you tell someone you are sick and he feels like now I can't give you a handshake because he sick. But we thank God, through sensitization, education, and these seminars, people are now enlightened about HIV. And we accept them as our brothers and sisters.

Except in a few cases, there are a few cases when you are sick, your family runs away from you. They separate you, they keep you in a separate room."[136] The above observation, made by a sheikh who works as part of a consortium of Islamic leaders addressing stigma and discrimination in Nairobi offers a forthright yet vexing picture of how the disease has historically been conjured in the Muslim imagination. The stigma associated with AIDS is so powerful that, above, we see that families turn their back on relatives and loved ones living with infection. As the culmination of both the crisis of education and the crisis of prevention, stigmatization of those living with HIV and AIDS in Kenya is a systemic problem, one that mandates an aggressive campaign to combat the negative effects of discrimination.

This is because, historically, the basic facts regarding the etiology of AIDS and modes of transmission were misunderstood, judged from a moral perspective, and were fomented by various religious leaders throughout the city leading to further entrenched misconceptions about the epidemic. "One of the biggest or hardest things we've had is this issue of stigma. First, when HIV/AIDS information came to us we were taught that HIV is a disease of the wrongdoers—only people who do promiscuous activities like prostitution, or lesbianism," stated one Muslim physician about the challenges of destigmatization. "They were the ones who are gay—and people like that, who are perceived from the point of religious leaders that they are wrongdoers. That information—that first information which we received—has an impact on the programs up to now."[137]

This medical doctor sees stigma as a major issue in the overall Muslim strategy to counter the AIDS epidemic in Kenya. Within this moralistic view, the focus looks at the individual's actions that led to disease transmission which assumes some ethical judgment of the person living with the infection. And perhaps one of the most problematic aspects of stigma is that it is an intangible dimension of the epidemic—though one with disastrous consequences for those toward whom it is directed.

Interestingly, one of the major factors leading to stigma, at least as a matter of externality, is the Kenyan government's initiatives in addressing the disease during the early days of the AIDS crisis. As with any structural problem, there is the consistent need for sustained effort—from both the national government and from international donors to address the impact of the AIDS epidemic as it relates to stigma and discrimination. "The government has done some efforts to address the issues of HIV. First, through the declaration as a disaster. That was the effective way through which donors were able to fund the activities related to HIV and AIDS," offered one young Muslim official. "But at the moment, there are no funds to target the infected in the community. There is a case whereby people for the community were fundraising for ARV's. So the effort is going down as time goes by."[138]

While at first glance this account of government funding might not seem to deal directly with the crisis of stigma in dealing with AIDS, the unintended consequence of the lack of continued funding does in fact have negative consequences in the area of destigmatization. “It’s a problem. It’s a problem. Because if it all we have sensitization trainings that at the end people are able to come out. Once you have already targeting these people, you’ve known their HIV status,” the subject observed. “Then what next? Are you able to sustain, maybe have a sustainability strategy? Now, for those on ARV’s, for example, are they able to continue having ARV’s with no funds for the activities related to HIV? So it’s a challenge.”[139] While not an obvious corollary of funding constraints, the Islamic official brings up a very compelling point—what of the imams who have attended sensitization training, and what of those that did not have the opportunity due to lack of funding? What of those living positively in the Muslim community, making known their status, and what of those individuals who maintain a moralistic view toward how people contracted the disease? This is not even to mention the issue of access to ARV’s which entails both treatment and justice.

What emerges is a complex web of factors that lead to deep theological questions concerning how to address and eventually ease the stigma directed toward people living with HIV and AIDS in Nairobi. On the topic of treatment and ARV’s in relation to stigma, whereas the disease can be managed through effective treatment regimens, there is to date no known cure for HIV or AIDS. And where stigma is often attributed to external forces such as popular opinion, there is also the dimension of self-stigma for those Muslims living with infection and how they perceive themselves. This self-stigma can lead to various coping mechanisms—among them denial, silence, anger, self-loathing, and despair.

In terms of treatment, the desperation associated with self-stigma may lead the infected Muslim to seek out alternative forms of treatment, and in some cases, faith healing. “You see, for example, there are issues of faith healing. Ok—I believe that if God wills, anything is possible. But then the way people are doing it, you see in every area there are con men. You get con men who are engineers, con men who are pharmacists,” said one Muslim health official. “The other day if you saw in the news three or four days ago, there are raids in certain parts of Nairobi and there are so many pharmacists and chemists which are fake. They didn’t have proper documentation, they are not graduates in their fields.”[140] Reminiscent of the *Hadith* cited in the section on education as *kairos*, that God has appointed a remedy for every illness—those, in some iterations of this *Hadith*, it concludes with the admonition, to not use anything unlawful as proscribed in the Qur’an.[141]

This verse helps to clarify the above account since this treatment is outside of the prescribed medical treatment recommended and advocated for by most sheikhs and imams in Nairobi. However, this deception is not limited exclusively to medicine. Indeed, there are even priests and imams who claim to be able to cure people from the disease. The leader stated further regarding stigma and despair, "even in the sector, the religious sector, it's also—there are also con men who have also entered. People who have never studied theology, they don't know anything about it. They just impose themselves, and then they go for easy money. If somebody is desperate, you tell anything to that person and he believes."[142] This social development of consulting faith healers provides some insight into the lengths that people will go—physically, spiritually, geographically, and even monetarily—to abate the self-stigma of an HIV diagnosis. Self-stigma, then, is one of the multidimensional though interrelated dimensions of the crisis of stigma in the Muslim population in Nairobi.

One other area of stigma that can lead those living with infection to despair is the general belief among Muslims that the diagnosis of HIV carries some judgment in terms of morality since it is most notably associated with sexuality. "Initially it was very bad because, just like in other communities, people associated HIV and AIDS with fornication and adultery," lamented one imam with offices in Nairobi. "And therefore, in Islam there is a verse that says 'Do not come close to committing adultery.' "[143] Such an instinctive reaction—that people became infected with HIV through fornication and adultery—manifests a facile understanding of the disease many sheikhs and imams had been promoting, thus making destigmatization efforts significantly more complicated.

Because of this generalization about disease transmission, there has historically been a dimension of denial surrounding the epidemic as well as stigmatization and discrimination from within the broader Islamic community in Nairobi. The subsequent silence of those infected stems from the fear of going public with their infection status, which might lead to lower prevalence rates among the Muslim population. In several studies, researchers—both secular and religious—have concluded that the seroprevalence rate among the Muslim population of Eastern Africa is strikingly lower than their Christian counterparts, and along the coastal regions and island archipelagos have even lower infection rates.[144]

The science seems to corroborate the fact that the relatively wholesome, local Islamic lifestyle does not lend itself to HIV and AIDS infection to the same degree as other religious groups.[145] However, where this statistic is correlative, it most certainly is not causative. As one Muslim respondent unabashedly admitted, "Stigma and discrimination makes a problem—for the researchers, some of the research you can see some of the Muslim areas recording low prevalence to HIV and AIDS. So many people think there's nothing, HIV and AIDS are not in the Muslim community. But they have to look at the factors, factors that maybe refers to zero prevalence to HIV."[146] This is a remarkable assertion, that the recorded rates within the Muslim population in Kenya might not be as accurate as once thought. While there are variable and statistical variations, the subject stated, "But there are some factors to research. It might be that they are very infected, but due to the stigma associated with disclosure, then people don't turn out for the research. So you end up with the wrong data, wrong data for the entire thing," stated the subject.[147]

This is a very important point in terms of the widespread effect of stigma on how the Kenyan Muslims perceive the disease—particularly since one element of stigma involves, at some basic level, behavior modification or the perception of a standard of acceptable behavior. To admit openly that someone has contracted the disease even now in some Muslim communities is to be met with discrimination and disdain.[148] It would certainly follow that when research is being done on the topic of AIDS and Islam, those infected would not seek to be publicly recognized for fear of judgment and other forms of social repercussions. Such a development presents a particularly troublesome obstacle for those engaged in stigma mitigation to overcome, since inaccurate reporting about infection rates may prove self-reinforcing—that the actual infection rate is artificially low because those with infection do not speak out due to stigma.

This does uphold the impression that HIV is not as much of a crisis for Kenyan Muslims, creating a dangerous precedent for those at risk who might mistakenly believe that AIDS is not a Muslim problem. The roots and reach of stigma toward PLWHA in Nairobi have served to undermine efforts toward empowering these Kenyans, making it appear infection is not something that Muslims should worry about. Not only does this perception of HIV engender future stigmatization, but other-izing behavior can also be attributed to nationalistic differences between Islamic groups living throughout the country. "And right now, actually, the stigma is very high within the Somali community—especially those who still live within their own enclaves," asserted one imam. "So they will not say that other people, will, should. . . . But they believe that 'we' cannot. Jut like before when Muslims believed, 'No, this disease is for those people who have committed adultery, fornication'—Somalis still believe that."[149]

Since Kenya shares a porous northern border with Somalia, there is a sizeable Somali population living within the geographic borders of Kenya, with one of the largest concentrations in Nairobi.[150] While this observation does show the promise that Kenyan Muslims are moving away from moral judgmentalism and stigma toward people with HIV and AIDS, it demonstrates a degree of other-izing behavior examined in the previous chapter—that some Kenyan Muslims believe the Somalis are using stigma to maintain a unified identity "within their own enclave." Still, it is notable that there are varying degrees of the effects of stigma within Islam in Kenya, not only on the individual but also collectively. However, as stigma aims both consciously and unconsciously to regulate behavior, it also involves a shift in focus over time since, as a behavioral issue, "any behavior is a process."[151]

Consequently, changing how people infected with HIV are viewed by the larger Muslim society in Nairobi necessarily involves a process of changing behavior. When coupled with the widespread belief that AIDS is not as severe among the Muslim population, this belief marks a movement away from the era of disease exceptionalism which raises its own concerns. Echoing the lasting impact of stigma and the belief that available treatment makes the medical condition manageable, one subject said that AIDS among the Muslim population of Nairobi, "doesn't receive as much attention as it did before. It's a common thing. We know, we know about it, we know how to prevent. And so, people who are there they get the disease, they live with it, there is treatment. So it's becoming an ordinary thing."[152]

This common misconception—that the AIDS epidemic in Kenya is no longer a crisis—has just as much to do with stigma as it does with prevention and education since stigma creates an unattainable standard of behavior for every person in the community. Those infected fear revealing their status due to moralistic and familial reprisals. Operating under the mistaken assumption that the epidemic is no longer a crisis can lead to an increase in infection rates, as Muslims fail to accept that there remain very physiological human elements of disease transmission—from accidental exposure in hospitals and barber stops to engaging in extra-marital affairs to IDU. Irrespective of religious affiliation, there are numerous modes of disease transmission and to overlook the urgency of the matter is to potentially place one's self in the way of harm.

On behavioral processes affected by stigma, the Muslim medical doctor acknowledged, "Muslims believe that if you don't correct a wrong in society the good and the bad will also be affected. So that initial idea that discriminating against those who were infected has now shifted to a much more accommodative situation, that some who are also innocent could be affected by this problem. So currently there is accepting of the situation, there is a merciful approach to those who are infected."[153] The admission that there is no identifiable at-risk group within the Muslim community—and that anyone can contract the disease, even those innocent of any moral infraction—marks a shift in how stigma is understood.

Reflecting on the crossroads between religion and medicine, the doctor points to the shift from the crisis of stigma to what he sees nowadays as more openness to people living with the virus, stating "the fact that now we have kind of effective antiretroviral treatment that goes with—and people seem to be able to live longer—then it's much more tolerated really, that people can quietly go on with their work whether they are HIV positive. So the disease is becoming a little more—not totally acceptable—but somehow people can live with it."[154] This sentiment is in itself fairly constitutive of the crisis of stigma, that even though ARV's are available in Nairobi, the disease is tolerated so long as those living with the disease are quiet about their status.

Even full acceptance of the disease today is not fully supported by all sectors of the Muslim community and stigma remains a problem. This is in part because the disease is, in the words of the Muslim physician, "manageable. It's not a crisis anymore."[155] This is a very troubling viewpoint, since if the AIDS epidemic in Nairobi is no longer a crisis, then by extension the virus is no longer a problem that people feel the need to address. This dismissive logic poses serious risk for the infected Islamic population of Kenya's capital since silence breeds disease. To combat this mistaken belief that AIDS is no longer a crisis, a *kairos* of destigmatization is necessary.

Destigmatization as *Kairos*

> Ok. The good thing or the positive side of it is that—a few years ago, there is a lot of stigma and people thought that this is not our problem, it was not our disease, so on and so forth. But now, out of a lot of sensitization and education and information sharing, there is a lot of good response from the community—in the sense of them also being informed, one. Two, from that informed position they are able to integrate. For example, widows whose husbands or widowers whose spouses have died out of HIV/AIDS, we have been able to empower them with some microfinance projects so that they can help themselves. The other side regards the orphans as a result of HIV/AIDS. Without stigma, an orphan is an orphan as a result of HIV/AIDS, or as a result of their parents died from accident, or any other disease—cancer also, so forth. We are able to habilitate them with other orphans. Then, on the other side, is we are able to open some VCT centers inside our mosque complex or Islamic institutions. So those are very positive steps we've taken.[156]

This broad overview of efforts directed at destigmatization in the Muslim community in Nairobi indicates a pivotal shift in the historical crisis of stigma attached to people infected with HIV and AIDS. Realistically, it identifies three areas of practical response stemming from stigma mitigation—ownership of the disease that affects the Islamic population; positive living through empowerment of those negatively affected by the epidemic; and finally, moving past the era of AIDS exceptionalism that has historically drawn a negative focus on those living with infection and their families.

The lasting effect of these strategic aims among Muslims in Nairobi demonstrates that real steps are being taken in the various sectors of HIV and AIDS destigmatization. Practically and theologically there has been a shift in how people perceive and accept people living with infection as a conceptual movement from crisis to *kairos*. For example, one Muslim leader attested that, "HIV is a condition that can affect anyone in the community. It does not discriminate based on religion, gender, and then color or race. HIV is a condition that can affect anyone in the society."[157] This belief, which clearly illustrates that there is a change in how the epidemic is viewed from a Muslim perspective, can be seen as informed by the religious community asserting ownership over the disease as well as a movement past the idea that AIDS is exceptional. For, if the disease doesn't discriminate based on ethnic or social factors, how can the Islamic population discriminate against people living with the virus in Nairobi?

One other obvious dimension motivating stigma mitigation efforts is that Muslims working in this particular field have begun to propose notions of the disease that look to the person's inherent dignity, that they reflect some divine essence that needs to be acknowledged—similar to the concept of man being created in the *imago dei* in Christianity. Reflecting on the developments that constitute the *kairos* of opportunity in destigmatization, one sheikh looked to the positive effect of such efforts, saying, "I can say it has been effective. We have seen positive things. We have seen people who used to know different things about HIV now changing their minds. People who used to run away from sick people, now they approach them, they talk to them, they share like World Cup—they can share that. Before that it was something impossible. There is some change."[158]

With this practical account, something apparently as simple as watching a soccer match with someone infected was historically problematic due to the presence of stigma and fear. Now, by owning the disease and admitting that it is an Islamic problem, the community in Nairobi changes and stands alongside their infected brothers and sisters, not only as Muslims but fundamentally as humans. Of course, within the broader religious community, the sheikh and imam are integral in promoting this idea and maintaining a consistent message, which itself can prove problematic. Due to their position as religious and social leaders, Islamic officials stand at the crossroads of a dynamic practical and theological change concerning stigma. "Because you see, the religious leaders are the role models to the community. Then on the other side, there are some who are stigmatized. So there's also need to target the religious leaders," signaled one imam on the importance of religious leaders. "Not all of them are able to talk about HIV. Some can be open, talk about HIV and then some, some are not open. So there is also need for them to be targeted. Because if they are targeted, then they can be very effective to the community because they are role models."[159]

Such a theologically, medically, and practically difficult discourse carries with it its own troubles, not least of all how imams and sheikhs address the issue of stigma in the *madrasas* and mosques. Further, as the officials presiding over the burials of those who have succumbed to opportunistic infection as the result of AIDS, Islamic religious leaders are important figures in addressing stigma and changing how the community perceives the disease.

"But slowly, when people started understanding the HIV and AIDS transmission, then they started appreciating the need for intervention. Now we have, we can see some imams who are actively advocating through the pulpit, fighting against HIV and AIDS, sensitizing people on HIV and AIDS," one imam noted on the influence of the imam in historically dealing with stigma. "Now, when people die, it's not a secret that information will go out—that maybe they were infected by HIV and AIDS. Initially they would say it's heart attack, it's cancer, whatever. But now, it is improving. Not as much as in the Christian world though, we still have our own stigma. But *Al-ḥamdo lellāh*, it's improving."[160] This account addresses popular conceptions of how Muslim and Christian efforts have differed, the imam does admit that there has been a change in even the vocabulary that Islamic leaders use in speaking about the disease and those infected.

This "improvement" signals a shift also for how the religious leaders can serve to transform the hearts and minds of their congregations. The imam remarked on influencing common policy and rituals in everyday life in Nairobi:

> Everybody is using gloves. Everybody is using gloves. Ok that's one. Two, there is of course also within that, of course the imams will talk when they are presiding over the burial, they will say that of course there are many things affecting us. They use the opportunity to talk to people about HIV and AIDS. And of course not saying that the diseased were affected by HIV and AIDS. But we just want to caution young people that we are living our own values and we are getting into some of those things. So for me, I think people are becoming a little more open talking about HIV and AIDS. People are confessing that they are positive, it's no longer embarrassing for some people. I know quite a number myself of friends and relatives are really open about it and they just tell you, "I am positive." In this office we handle people who are looking for spouses. And the people are coming and tell us, "I am looking for a spouse who is HIV positive like me. Because I tested positive." So, because of course eventually when we are filling our forms, we tell them that they will have to go for HIV test, but many of them have told us—have disclosed it without even going through the forms. So there is some level of awareness.[161]

The imam, working with affiliate bodies such as SUPKEM and KCI serves both a religiously and dramatically practical role. Speaking of values and talking to people about HIV and AIDS can be seen to fill a pastoral function within the Islamic community—easing discrimination and embarrassment.

Yet, another dimension of the epidemic in human terms is that imams are continually being asked to serve in the position as mediator between those who are infected and those looking for spouses. This is perhaps one of the most powerful aspects of the *karios* of stigma mitigation—that after accepting that the disease does affect a portion of Muslims, Islamic leaders can work out a way to serve the person as a person, including helping them find love and start a family even with AIDS infection. Following from this, the imam and sheikh in Nairobi can empower people living with the virus not only providing material support—such as the micro-financing projects cited at the beginning of this section—but also in terms of pastoral and social support.

In one anecdote, the imam spoke of a support group for eighty Muslim couples who are living with HIV and AIDS. "And they are actually couples, husband and wife. Very few among them are discordant couples. All of them, most of them are actually both infected. We have them and we provide some support, we also call it social support and material support when it comes to that kind of need. And they are ok, they live amongst their own people and we don't see anything," said the imam. Such a practical observation and assessment of the lives of Muslim couples who are living with infection yet striving to live positively displays a depth of humanity that ennobles those working in the area of stigma reduction. This is belied, however, by the fact that social stigma still exists regarding the epidemic within the Muslim community—both from the leadership and from the laity.

The imam continued, "We still have that stigma among some people, we have the stigma. But the fact that cancer seems to be taking more lives than HIV and AIDS people are appreciating that, 'Eh, you know sometimes you'd rather have HIV and AIDS than cancer because cancer will finish you within a couple of months or years, but HIV and AIDS is managed.' "[162] This belief that the epidemic is manageable—while it does lend emphasis to the view that AIDS is no longer a crisis—also marks a shift in perception that to be diagnosed with the disease is not necessarily a death sentence. Medically, the physical condition and theologically the stigma attendant to the condition are treatable.

This change begins with an internal reconceptualization for the sheikhs and imams that minister to the Muslim population in Nairobi, who serve to sensitize people by talking about important issues facing the population from the pulpit and arranging gatherings at the community halls to stage seminars to help Muslims familiarize themselves with the technical aspects of the virus. Specific to stigma reduction is speaking to and reaching out to those living with infection, who themselves are often living in a state of self-stigmatization:

> Well, in terms of those affected and living with HIV and AIDS, for me it's just to encourage them to not give up. People are born without limbs, and they become the best in terms of giving to society. So, if you've been blessed to have HIV and AIDS, just take advantage of the situation and give back to society, give back to God what God expects of you as a person. So just to encourage that there are more worse aliments than HIV and AIDS. There's cancer, there is Ebola—there are quite a lot of worse ailments. So people should not see HIV as a very bad ailment. Nobody of course would want to be

> in that situation, nobody would want to be on medication throughout your entire life. But we know that there are many people who are on medication throughout their entire lives and they are not suffering from HIV and AIDS. So it's to encourage them, open up, talk to people about it, encourage—use your situation, use yourself as an example—and encourage people to really just be good human beings.[163]

These remarks get to the very human, practical dimension of the destigmatization efforts by Muslim leaders in Nairobi, that while there is a relative scale of diseases, ailments, and afflictions, coming to terms with the religious and physical dimensions of being human can sometimes be one of the largest practical challenges to stigma.

Nevertheless, Islamic leaders are using their positions to be agents of empowerment so that, in all areas of life, people living with the disease, their families and friends can "really just be good human beings." From the perspective of the Islamic leadership, one of the most impactful elements of stigma mitigation is that, while informed by Qur'ānic teaching, these individuals are part of the overarching Muslim community. The epidemic therefore intimately affects them as human beings. Often, the imam's interaction with the virus takes on an all too personal tone, as with the sheikh who spoke of the *janazah* burial ceremony and prayer for those Muslims who have died. "Of course. Even I myself, I've seen more than once from my own family with my uncle dying because of this disease," he confirmed. "And with . . . more than 10 cases I have witnessed imams perform the *janazah* prayer because someone has died of HIV. Some of them are all our own family members, like me—I have three of them who have died from the disease. So its not something you forget."[164]

This striking comment offers an intimate yet terribly realistic assessment of what it is like to be a religious leader living in Kenya through the HIV and AIDS epidemic. Marking the shift from AIDS as exceptional to empowering those living with infection is a distinct change in attitude, particularly in terms of stigma from the Islamic perspective. In this case, there is extensive overlap between the three fields selected for analysis in this chapter—prevention, education, and destigmatization—and yet, stigma is so pervasive that it affects even the way people perceive familial bonds and kinship ties.

One of the salient elements of Islamic efforts at destigmatization in Nairobi is that the disease is viewed as a condition that affects the physical human person, one that influences human behavior as well as human relationships, both family and intimate. The movement from crisis to *kairos* in stigma mitigation involves the challenge of shame and discrimination being transformed into the opportunity for openness and acceptance of the person negatively affected by the virus. "In past years, it was like a shame to say 'My brother died of HIV.' But nowadays things have changed, because people have been sensitized, because people have been educated about HIV," noted one member of the Kenyan Council of Imams on coming to terms with AIDS—and the progression from shame to openness. "Even some of them, they just come out openly—'I am HIV positive.' And you just discuss with people, 'I was infected in this way.' So things have changed from that desire of hiding things, now people are being open, 'I am sick. I tell you I am sick.' So, things have changed, not like before."[165]

This shift from silence and denial to openness and acceptance signals an important development for the Muslim population in Nairobi, that by self-consciously admitting that someone is living with infection, initiatives in destigmatization, education, and prevention can take on a completely new form and mandate leading to a markedly more positive response to the epidemic in Kenya. And, as noted above, one of the most effective ways to change how people perceive the disease is through reformulating standard Islamic teaching in new ways which look past judgment and moralism to better understand the basic human condition as contingent on the *tawhīd* and unicity of God:

> Ok, whoever is infected by HIV, then what they should do, they should accept themselves as a sick person. And they should accept the fact that he is affected with HIV, and he should not make effort of spreading it, saying "Because I've got it, now I have to give it." They should try to live in a positive way, taking good care of themselves and taking good care of the people living with them. Not just decide, "Ok now that I'm infected, now I just live my own life," and take off over there. Then they should know it's just a test for them because we as Muslims, we believe that whenever you're sick, then it's a test from God. If you just believe it is from Allah, from now until the day you die, then you get more tests. In Islam, we have been taught that whenever you are sick, whenever you are going through any difficulties, believe that it is only Allah that can save you. So my advice for them is that it is just have patience for now. Let them try to accept who they are, "Ok I've been infected. *Al-ḥamdo lellāh*, it is from Allah." And you try to live a positive life, not to harm anybody with the disease and just believe that Allah will provide. That is how to live.[166]

Though this view of the virus as a test for the Muslim faithful can lend itself to a moralistic reading into the disease transmission, it is a useful Islamic teaching for how people should view and interact with those living with infection—rather than being silent and denying that it is a problem, HIV infection as a testing circumstance for the human presents a new way to understand the disease, as a challenge that Muslims can confront, treat, and eventually overcome, representing the *kairos* of the appointed time for God's activity. This is equally true of stigma that humans direct toward those who have historically been treated as outsiders because of their infection status. This means that, as a community of faithful believers, Muslims in Nairobi can, should, and indeed must work together to eradicate stigma shown to those living with infection so that they may take part in the common good of society. Islamic leaders are thus called to uphold the inherent dignity of those negatively affected by the epidemic and serving as instruments of social change to realize the *kairos* of stigma mitigation.

CONCLUSION: "THIS THING HAS NO BOUNDARIES."

Islamic efforts in prevention, education, and destigmatization toward the AIDS epidemic in Nairobi are varied, as the subjects in this chapter offer a broad range of views on each of the three strategic objectives and their efficacy. That this chapter employed the sociological and theological distinction of a movement from crisis to *kairos* merits consideration once more, since it offers a distinction between HIV as both a sociohistorical event and a theological matter for consideration. Thus, the epidemic in Nairobi inhabits a rather interesting practical and conceptual intersection that engages issues that involve the whole person, both spiritually and physical, both body and soul.

"Ok, we might differ on opinions. But there are some, but minority, who feel that these things should not be discussed in the mosque. It is a shame to mention HIV on the pulpit. But the majority of the imams, they came to realize that this thing has no boundaries," a sheikh involved in HIV and AIDS outreach and advocacy through the Kenyan Council of Imams forthrightly acknowledged. "You are forced to talk about it, because when somebody starts dying from HIV you begin getting AIDS orphans from HIV. So we have no other option but in discussing this issue. There is some opposition, of course there is."[167]

This assessment treats one of the major issues facing the work being done to combat the spread of HIV among the Muslim leadership. That is, even with very diverse opinions on prevention, education, and stigma mitigation—each of which entail historical, cultural, social, ethic, economic, governmental, and theological factors. Due to the urgency of the AIDS epidemic in Nairobi, Islamic officials are compelled to address the underlying issues associated with HIV and AIDS in their own communities—oftentimes by using Islamic teaching and theological traditions.

And this sheikh is right, that AIDS has no boundaries and so everyone—both Muslim and Catholic, clergy and laity—are affected by this virus in markedly similar and yet personally different ways. This understanding of the virus reaches past the epidemic in Kenya as a historical crisis confronting one particular social milieu to a religious understanding that offers itself instead as an opportunity for leaders to come together to be representatives of God's action here on earth. Because of the similarities between Catholic and Islamic practical and religious activity in responding to HIV in Nairobi, the next chapter offers a comparative theological analysis of the interreligious traditions of mercy, hospitality, and justice operative in the three strategic efforts from within both Sunni Islam and African Catholicism.

NOTES

1. The opening quotation was taken from Stephen Hirtenstein and Martin Notcutt, *Divine Sayings: 101 Hadith Qudsi* (Oxford, UK: Anqa Publishing, 2008), 75.
2. Freeman-Grenville, "Al-Mas'udi: The Ivory Trade," 17.
3. David Whitehouse,"East Africa and the Maritime Trade of the Indian Ocean, AD 800–1500," in *Islam in East Africa: New Sources*, ed. Biancamaria Amoretti (Rome, Italy: International Colloquium, 2001), 418.
4. Freeman-Grenville, "Al-Mas'udi: The Ivory Trade," 16–17.
5. Ibid., 102–3.
6. Ibid., 193–94.
7. Becker, *Becoming Muslim in Mainland Tanzania*, 46–50.
8. Randall L. Pouwels, *Horn and Crescent: Cultural Exchange and Traditional Islam on the East African Coast, 800–1900* (New York: Cambridge University Press, 1987), 100.
9. Ibid.
10. Becker, *Becoming Muslim in Mainland Tanzania*, 93.
11. Ibid., 92–98.
12. Ibid.
13. Pouwels, *Horn and Crescent*, 147–49; 195–97.
14. Becker, *Becoming Muslim in Mainland Tanzania*, 229–33.
15. Ibid., 209.
16. Moses Oketch and Caine Rolleston, "Policies on Free Primary Secondary Education in East Africa: Retrospect and Prospect," *Journal of Research in Education* 31 (2007): 131–32.
17. Johannes Svensson, " 'Muslims Have Instructions': HIV/AIDS, Modernity and Islamic Religious Education in Kisumu, Kenya," in *AIDS and Religious Practice in Africa*, 196.
18. Becker, *Becoming Muslim in Mainland Tanzania*, 143.
19. Ibid., 173
20. Ibid., 148.
21. Ibid.
22. Pouwels, *Horn and Crescent*, 89.
23. Becker, *Becoming Muslim in Mainland Tanzania*, 137–38; 141–43.
24. Derek Nurse and Thomas Spear, *The Swahili: Reconstructing the History and Language of an African Society, 800–1500* (Philadelphia: University of Pennsylvania Press, 1985), 4. A similar trend occurred in the Zionist churches of South Africa. See Peter Knox, SJ, *AIDS, Ancestors, and Salvation* (Nairobi, Kenya: Paulines Publications Africa, 2005), and Isak Niehaus, "Leprosy of a Deadlier Kind: Christian Conceptions of AIDS in the South African Lowveld," in *AIDS and Religious Practice in Africa*, eds. Felicitas Becker and P. Wenzel Geissler.
25. Personal Interview—Nairobi, Kenya, 6.17.14; 6.11.14.
26. Becker, *Becoming Muslim in Mainland Tanzania*, 8.
27. Bénézet Bujo, "Community Ethics," in *AIDS in Africa,* 69; Knox, *AIDS, Ancestors, and Salvation*, 95.
28. Becker, *Becoming Muslim in Mainland Tanzania*, 148.
29. Eds. Molefi Kete Asante and Abu S. Abarry, "Jomo Kenyatta, Religion and Ancestor Worship" in *African Intellectual Heritage: A Book of Sources*, eds. Molefi Kete Asante and Abu S. Abarry (Philadelphia: Temple University Press, 1996), 88–89.
30. Becker, *Becoming Muslim in Mainland Tanzania*, 171.
31. Janet McIntosh, *The Edge of Islam: Power, Personhood, and Ethnoreligious Boundaries on the Kenyan Coast* (Durham, NC: Duke University Press, 2009), 196.
32. Ibid.

33. Becker, *Becoming Muslim in Mainland Tanzania*, 159.
34. Ibid.
35. Ibid.
36. Ibid. 160.
37. Ibid.
38. McIntosh, *The Edge of Islam*, 197.
39. Ibid., 196.
40. Becker, *Becoming Muslim in Mainland Tanzania*, 159.
41. Ibid.
42. Ibid., 304.
43. Ibid., 159.
44. Muhammad ibn Abd ‘Allah al-Khatb al-Tibriz, *Mishkat al-Masabih*, Vol. II, trans. James Robson (Islamabad, Pakistan: Orentalia Arts Ltd., 1999), 948.
45. Becker, *Becoming Muslim in Mainland Tanzania*, 159.
46. CIA, “Africa—Kenya,” 3.
47. Svensson, “ ‘Muslims Have Instructions’: HIV/AIDS, Modernity and Islamic Religious Education in Kisumu, Kenya,” 193.
48. Personal Interview—Nairobi, Kenya, 6.11.14.
49. Svensson, “ ‘Muslims Have Instructions’: HIV/AIDS, Modernity and Islamic Religious Education in Kisumu, Kenya,” 192.
50. Adam Ashforth, “An Epidemic of Witchcraft? The Implications of AIDS for the Post-Apartheid State,” *African Studies* 61.1 (2002): 121–43.
51. Personal Interview—Nairobi, Kenya, 7.23.14.
52. Ibid.
53. CIA, “Africa—Kenya,” 3.
54. Personal Interview—Nairobi, Kenya, 7.23.14.
55. Ibid.
56. See Abdhalah Kasiira Ziraba, Catherine Kyobutungi, and Eliya Msiyaphazi Zulu, “Fatal Injuries in the Slums of Nairobi and Their Risk Factors: Results from a Matched Case-Control Study,” *Journal of Urban Health: Bulletin of the New York Academy of Medicine* 88, suppl. 2 (2011). The result for those who imbibe such drinks can lead to inexpensive intoxication, but with the lack of standardization in the past, as this subject notes, side effects can include illness, blindness, and in the most extreme cases, death.
57. Adam Otieno, “Drug Abuse in Kisumu Town, Western Kenya,” *African Journal of Food, Agriculture, Nutrition, and Development* 9:3 (2009), 1–10.
58. Personal Interview—Nairobi, Kenya, 6.11.14.
59. Personal Interview—Nairobi, Kenya, 6.19.14.a.
60. Personal Interview—Nairobi, Kenya, 6.17.14.
61. Ibid.
62. Ibid.
63. Personal Interview—Nairobi, Kenya, 7.3.14.
64. Ibid.
65. Personal Interview—Nairobi, Kenya, 6.11.14.
66. Ibid.
67. Personal Interview—Nairobi, Kenya, 6.12.14.
68. Ibid.
69. Personal Interview—Nairobi, Kenya, 6.17.14.
70. Ibid.
71. Ibid.
72. Personal Interview—Nairobi, Kenya, 6.12.14.
73. Personal Interview—Nairobi, Kenya, 6.19.14.a.
74. Personal Interview—Nairobi, Kenya, 6.11.14.
75. Ibid.
76. Peter B. Gray, “HIV and Islam: Is HIV Prevalence Lower among Muslims?” *Social Science and Medicine* 58.9 (2004): 1751–56; Jamal Nasir Khan, Sukhmeet Singh Panesar, Abdul Rashid Gatrad, and Aziz Sheikh, “The Cross, the Crescent, and the Contagion: Ecologi-

cal Study of the Association between Religious Affiliation to Christianity and Islam, and Adult Prevalence of HIV/AIDS in Africa," *Journal of the Islamic Medical Association of South Africa* 12.1 (2005): 17–18.

77. Ibid.
78. See Badri, "The AIDS Crisis: An Islamic Perspective," 28–35.
79. Personal Interview—Nairobi, Kenya, 6.11.14.
80. Ibid.
81. Personal Interview—Nairobi, Kenya, 6.12.14.
82. Ibid.
83. Ibid.
84. Personal Interview—Nairobi, Kenya, 6.11.14.
85. Ibid.
86. Ibid.
87. Ibid.
88. Personal Interview—Nairobi, Kenya, 6.19.14.a.
89. Personal Interview—Nairobi, Kenya, 6.17.14.
90. Ibid.
91. Ibid.
92. Personal Interview—Nairobi, Kenya, 6.19.14.a.
93. Ibid.
94. Ibid.
95. Ibid.
96. Personal Interview—Nairobi, Kenya, 6.19.14.b.
97. Personal Interview—Nairobi, Kenya, 6.18.14.
98. Personal Interview—Nairobi, Kenya, 6.12.14.
99. Ibid.
100. Ibid.
101. Ibid.
102. Personal Interview—Nairobi, Kenya, 6.19.14.a.
103. Personal Interview—Nairobi, Kenya, 6.12.14.
104. Ibid.
105. Personal Interview—Nairobi, Kenya, 6.17.14.
106. Ibid.
107. See Hansjörg Dilger, "Sexuality, AIDS and the Lures of Modernity: Reflexivity and Morality among Young People in Rural Tanzania." *Medical Anthropology* 22.1 (2003): 23–52; Paul Wenzel Geissler and Ruth Prince, *The Land Is Dying: Contingency, Creativity, and Conflict in Western Kenya* (Oxford, UK: Berghahn Books, 2010); David A. Goldenberg, *We Are All Brothers: The Suppression of Consciousness of Socio-Economic Differentiation in a Kenya Luo Lineage* (Ann Arbor, MI: University Microfilms, Int'l, 1982); Ruth Prince, "Christian Salvation and Luo Tradition: Arguments of Faith in a Time of Death in Western Kenya," in *AIDS and Religious Practice in Africa*, eds. Felicitas Becker and P. Wenzel Geissler.
108. Personal Interview—Nairobi, Kenya, 6.12.14.
109. Ibid.
110. Ibid.
111. Personal Interview—Nairobi, Kenya, 6.17.14.
112. Ibid.
113. Personal Interview—Nairobi, Kenya, 6.12.14.
114. Personal Interview—Nairobi, Kenya, 6.17.14.
115. Personal Interview—Nairobi, Kenya, 6.12.14.
116. Personal Interview—Nairobi, Kenya, 6.18.14.
117. Ibid.
118. Ibid.
119. Ibid.
120. Personal Interview—Nairobi, Kenya, 6.17.14.
121. Personal Interview—Nairobi, Kenya, 6.19.14.a.

122. As one sheikh cynically yet realistically noted, "If you keep on talking about [HIV and AIDS], some might feel that this guy has no other topic." Personal Interview—Nairobi, Kenya, 6.19.14.b.
123. Personal Interview—Nairobi, Kenya, 6.19.14.c.
124. Ibid.
125. Personal Interview—Nairobi, Kenya, 6.11.14.
126. Personal Interview—Nairobi, Kenya, 6.17.14. Collected elsewhere, the *Hadith*, Number 18 collected by Ibn al-Arabi, the Andalusian mystic and philosopher of the twelfth century, reads, " 'O child of Adam, I was sick, and you did not visit Me.' [The man] asks: 'My Lord, how could I visit you when you are the Lord of the universes?' He will reply, 'Did you not know that one of my servants was sick, and you did not visit him? Did you not know that if you had visited him, you would have found Me with him?'" God then goes on to challenge the believer in terms of whether he has fed or given drink to the hungry and thirsty, respectively. This *Hadith* highlights the interdependence of all humans, and how God's divine essence lives and is reflected within each of ourselves. Hirtenstein and Notcutt, *Divine Sayings*, 75.
127. Personal Interview—Nairobi, Kenya, 6.17.14.
128. Ibid.
129. Personal Interview—Nairobi, Kenya, 6.19.14.b.
130. Personal Interview—Nairobi, Kenya, 6.19.14.a.
131. Malik Badri writes about AIDS as God's punishment to humanity at length in his chapter, "The AIDS Crisis: An Islamic Perspective," in *Islam and AIDS*.
132. Personal Interview—Nairobi, Kenya, 6.19.14.c.
133. Personal Interview—Nairobi, Kenya, 6.17.14.
134. Ibid.
135. Personal Interview—Nairobi, Kenya, 6.19.14.a.
136. Personal Interview—Nairobi, Kenya, 6.19.14.b.
137. Personal Interview—Nairobi, Kenya, 6.12.14.
138. Personal Interview—Nairobi, Kenya, 6.18.14.
139. Ibid.
140. Personal Interview—Nairobi, Kenya, 6.12.14.
141. Cited in the *Mishkat al-Masabih*, "God has sent down both the disease and the cure, and He has appointed a cure for every disease, so treat yourselves medically, but use nothing unlawful." al-Tibriz, *Mishkat al-Masabih*, Vol. II, 948.
142. Personal Interview—Nairobi, Kenya, 6.12.14.
143. Personal Interview—Nairobi, Kenya, 6.17.14.
144. See Gray, "HIV and Islam: Is HIV Prevalence Lower among Muslims?"; Khan, Panesar, Gatrad, and Sheikh, "The Cross, the Crescent, and the Contagion: Ecological Study of the Association between Religious Affiliation to Christianity and Islam, and Adult Prevalence of HIV/AIDS in Africa"; Felicitas Becker, "Competing Explanations and Treatment Choices: Muslims, AIDS and ARVs in Tanzania," in *AIDS and Religious Practice in Africa*.
145. Becker, "Competing Explanations and Treatment Choices: Muslims, AIDS and ARVs in Tanzania," 156.
146. Personal Interview—Nairobi, Kenya, 6.18.14.
147. Ibid.
148. Svensson, "Muslims Have Instructions": HIV/AIDS, Modernity and Islamic Religious Education in Kisumu, Kenya," 191.
149. Personal Interview—Nairobi, Kenya, 6.17.14.
150. See Vincent Bakpetu Thompson, *Conflict in the Horn of Africa: The Kenya-Somali Border Problem 1941–2014* (Lanham, MD: UPA Publications, 2015).
151. Personal Interview—Nairobi, Kenya, 6.12.14.
152. Personal Interview—Nairobi, Kenya, 6.18.14.
153. Personal Interview—Nairobi, Kenya, 6.11.14
154. Ibid.
155. Ibid.
156. Personal Interview—Nairobi, Kenya, 6.12.14.
157. Personal Interview—Nairobi, Kenya, 6.18.14.

158. Personal Interview—Nairobi, Kenya, 6.19.14.b.
159. Personal Interview—Nairobi, Kenya, 6.18.14.
160. Personal Interview—Nairobi, Kenya, 6.17.14.
161. Ibid.
162. Ibid.
163. Personal Interview—Nairobi, Kenya, 6.18.14.
164. Personal Interview—Nairobi, Kenya, 6.19.14.b.
165. Personal Interview—Nairobi, Kenya, 6.19.14.c.
166. Personal Interview—Nairobi, Kenya, 6.19.14.a.
167. Personal Interview—Nairobi, Kenya, 6.19.14.b.

Chapter Three

"Mercy triumphs over judgment"

Comparative Theological Notions of Mercy, Hospitality, and Justice in the Lived Muslim and Catholic Response to HIV and AIDS in Kenya

INTRODUCTION AND PLAN FOR THE CHAPTER

Regarding the commonality between both Islam and Christianity and stemming from the research presented in the previous two chapters, this chapter posits that prevention efforts are motivated by the virtue of mercy; education is informed and motivated by the tradition of hospitality; and activity in the area of stigma mitigation is motivated by the call for social justice.[1] These three theological traditions and virtues empower religious leaders from both faith traditions to come to the aid of those negatively affected by HIV and AIDS. Mercy, hospitality, and justice are therefore intimately connected to the care of the human person being provided throughout Kenya within both Muslim and Catholic communities. When applied to the social reality of the AIDS epidemic in Nairobi, numerous related theological issues arise—prominent among them are questions related to salvation, redemption, pain, suffering, and ultimately death.

Consequently, Muslim and Catholic leaders within the field of health care face a peculiar challenge. On the one hand, they are called to attend to the spiritual well-being of those living with HIV infection. On the other hand, they are increasingly being charged with serving as the caretakers of the physical bodies of all those negatively affected by the virus. Indeed, Muslim and Catholic leaders who dedicate their lives to making sure effective health care and prevention are available to those living with infection embody the theological principle of mercy. Officials who enact curriculum reform to ensure that factually correct information is taught in the classroom and the *madrasa* are certainly serving in the tradition of interreligious hospitality. And finally, Muslims and Catholic working in the strategic efforts at stigma reduction seek to affirm the inherent dignity of the person living with AIDS through their pursuit of social justice.

The chapter proceeds in the following way. It begins with an analysis of the three areas of religious activity directed toward people infected with HIV and AIDS. However, where the previous chapters looked to the actual, lived response of Catholic and Muslim leaders in their own words, this chapter considers the corresponding theological notions for each of these areas of religious activity, identified as prevention and health care, education, and destigmatization, as an opportunity for comparison. The first major section identifies the common concept of mercy as operative in the practical area of prevention and health care, offering an extended comparative analysis from both the Catholic and Muslim perspective. The second major section, like the first, offers a comparative analysis of the theological tradition of hospitality as motivating the Muslim and Catholic strategic aims in education. Finally, the third major section comparatively identifies the theological virtue of justice as operative in both the Muslim and Catholic efforts at destigmatization since stigma seeks to diminish the basic integrity of the individual living with HIV infection in Nairobi.

The chapter concludes with a brief discourse on the comparative notions of mercy, hospitality, and justice as the foundation and opportunity for religious officials from both traditions, Catholic and Muslim, to reach past self-identifying religious boundaries in order to effectively meet the needs of all Kenyans living with infection so that they can provide care for the whole person in an interreligious manner.

PREVENTION, HEALTH CARE, AND MERCY

This section examines scriptural accounts of mercy in both the Bible and the *Hadith* traditions of the Prophet Muhammad which set the parameters of the comparative analysis. In identifying the salient elements of human acts of mercy in these sacred writings, the chapter then looks to why and how the theological virtue of mercy is critical in the interreligious efforts in AIDS prevention in Nairobi, which itself is inherently tied to health care. With this discussion, both Muslim and Catholic leaders attending to those infected with HIV and AIDS are driven to perform bodily acts of mercy toward not only the sick but for any marginalized member of society. Thus, as an actual interreligious response, priests and imams are compelled to develop and implement effective prevention programs within their own religious communities in Kenya's capital.

Mercy is, therefore, one of the most influential motivators for religious officials working in health care precisely because it is chiefly concerned with how to treat other human beings. While this will be made clear in subsequent sections, when humans engage in acts of mercy, they are doing so in relation to their fellow humans. Further, as scriptural accounts illuminate, when an individual performs a corporeal act of mercy for another, they are directing mercy toward God since the human is created in God's image. Similarly, though mercy belongs above all to God in the Islamic tradition—*Ar-Raḥmān*, "the All-Merciful" in Arabic—we as humans must reflect God's divine attributes through our own actions and interactions with other humans. Since within both religions, human nature is meant to reflect the divine, those performing merciful acts are making real the *kairos* of prevention within Muslim and Catholic communities in Nairobi.

Catholic Scripture and Mercy

Any discussion of mercy from the Catholic perspective should necessarily begin with an overview of the corporeal works of mercy found in the Gospel of Matthew 25:31–40. Matthew writes:

> When the Son of Man comes in his glory, and all the angels with him, then he will sit on the throne of his glory. All the nations will be gathered before him, and he will separate people one from another as a shepherd separates the sheep from the goats, and he will put the sheep at his right hand and the goats at the left. Then the king will say to those at his right hand, "Come, you that are blessed by my Father, inherit the kingdom prepared for you from the foundation of the world; for I was hungry and you gave me food, I was thirsty and you gave me something to drink, I was a stranger and you welcomed me, I was naked and you gave me clothing, I was sick and you took care of me, I was in prison and you visited me." Then the righteous will answer him, "Lord, when was it that we saw you hungry and gave you food, or thirsty and gave you something to drink? And when was it that we saw you a stranger and welcomed you, or naked and gave you clothing? And when was it that we saw you sick or in prison and visited you?" And the king will answer them, "Truly I tell you, just as you did it to one of the least of these who are members of my family, you did it to me."[2]

This list of corporeal works of mercy consists of seven injunctions qualifying the believing Christian from the non-believer—just as God will judge between the sheep and the goats. Since they are corporeal, by definition they deal with the human being as a matter of his or her immediate condition as human: Christians are called to provide food for the hungry and drink to the thirsty in order to nourish the body; they are directed to welcome the stranger and clothe the naked, which themselves do not sustain human survival, yet point to the interrelatedness humanity and the humility of the human condition; then finally, the last three corporeal works of mercy concern the isolation associated with being human—taking care of the sick, visiting the prisoner, and burying the dead.

Indeed, if the Christian faithful were not encouraged to attend to the sick, the imprisoned, and the dead—a responsibility that often falls on the immediate family—then the isolated human would remain alone. The Gospel of Matthew realistically offers an explicit blueprint for how Christians as followers of Jesus Christ should act—not only toward one another but also in general. It also sets the conditions on which the goats and sheep will be judged on the Day of Final Judgment.

When the same set of criteria for judgment are reformulated negatively immediately afterwards in the Gospel of Matthew, people are judged negatively for not giving food to the hungry, not giving drink to the thirsty—the "goats" are taken aback by their relative inactivity in performing these merciful works. "The parable of Matthew 25 is striking in that everyone is surprised by the judgment," writes noted Catholic ethicist Fr. James F. Keenan, SJ. "The sheep never realized that in feeding the hungry, they were feeding the king. Nor did the goats realize that by not visiting the sick, they were not visiting the Lord."[3]

This call for Christians to engage in works of mercy creates a very interesting dynamic, since those who perform them will be blessed and those that neglect them will be punished. While this seems at its very basis to be a matter of justice—especially in reference to judgment—these works can only be accomplished in relation to others. In showing mercy to those who are experiencing the human condition—the hungry, sick, and imprisoned—Christians can affirm that they are part of a social and historical community since they come to the aid of those in need, even if in the form of clothing or solace.

The human condition, therefore, exhibits both human and divine realities as both the performer of the merciful deeds and the recipient are part of God's own creation. Reflecting on the singular significance of mercy in Catholicism, Keenan continues, "Our entire theological tradition is expressed in terms of mercy, which I define as the willingness to enter into the chaos of others."[4] This definition of mercy—as entering into the chaotic experience of another person—is helpful in identifying mercy as the virtue corresponding to the Muslim and Catholic efforts in HIV and AIDS prevention in Nairobi. Since mercy does not operate in isolation, entering the chaos that is the life of another person necessitates that we pay heed to other people—both physiologically and socially. Stated differently, the moment you give food to a hungry person, or clothe the naked person, you automatically enter into the chaos and are a part of that person's and God's universe and narrative.

No matter how small, works of mercy have a reverberating impact, not only on the human person, but also on the divine. Even the Gospel of Matthew 25:40 illustrates this, with God stating, "Truly I tell you, just as you did it to one of the least of these who are members of my family, you did it to me."[5] This account very poignantly offers a three-fold analysis. First, the works of mercy are directed toward people who are in need and they draw you into the chaos of another living being. Second, performing the corporeal acts of mercy for others is as if you are performing them for God's self. Third, perhaps most important for this present research, performing the works of mercy draws you into an additional third level of chaos—that of family. However, this family is not though blood lineage and ancestry but rather it is one of confession that draws the human into the Christian family through right belief (orthodoxy, belief in the redemptive message of Jesus) and right action (orthopraxy, performing the acts of mercy).

Such a formulation of mercy demands that—since the Christian God is merciful—the Christian faithful themselves must also be merciful. On this topic, Rodney Stark writes regarding the early Christian community, "the corollary that *because* God loves humanity, Christians may not please God unless they *love one another* was even more incompatible with pagan convictions." He continues, "the truly revolutionary principle was that Christian love and charity must extend beyond the boundaries of family and even those of faith, to all in need."[6] From this familial dimension of the corporeal acts of mercy, there already exists a confessional "family" of believers, unified in the saving grace of Christ.

However, as noted previously, the merciful acts can be performed by complete strangers. As a matter of immediacy, the works of mercy create something of a family of love through Christ—but also one of necessity. When applied to the case of HIV and AIDS in Kenya, the result is something similar to what the early Christians experienced. That is, in contemporary Nairobi, there exists a complex web of identity—from ethnic, to cultural, to social, economic, political, and religious—that makes enunciating one monolithic identity impossible. For this reason, those Christians working in AIDS prevention are not only serving "with all those who in every place call on the name of our Lord Jesus Christ"—but on a much more general, human level, they are reinforcing the bonds that tie us all together as a basic human family.[7]

Mercy is therefore an incontestable element of prevention efforts in Kenya, as Catholic leaders deal daily with providing care to the physical organism that is the human person, particularly for those living with HIV and AIDS. Christian love, compassion, charity, and mercy "was the cultural basis for the revitalization of the Roman world groaning under a host of miseries."[8] In this way to every Christian, Rome resembles present day Nairobi which manifests many of the systematic issues that Christians—from the first century to today—are called to address. Chief among them are caring for those who are sick.

Specifically, as the works of mercy relate to the Catholic prevention efforts in Nairobi, one area of consideration is the plight of those living with the virus. As Matthew writes, one of the corporeal works of mercy is to care for the sick. This directive by its very nature entails caring for the human in a very physical sense, for the human as a living being is susceptible to illness. Germane to this section on prevention, the parable does not call doctors and nurses to provide care for the sick—presumably because it is their occupation to do so. Rather, the injunction is directed toward fellow Christians in a supererogatory fashion.

Even the wording itself is worth further consideration. The merciful work is not to cure the sick person, but rather to offer care for them. This observation is particularly true in Nairobi, since Catholic clergy seek to provide effective care—in the form of prevention programs and health care in general—for people living with infection. This is not in itself a recent development, at least not in terms of providing care to the human person—physically, theologically, spiritually, and morally—by the Catholic Church. Indeed, in his book *The Works of Mercy*, Fr. Keenan observes that, over the past two thousand years, the Church and members of the clergy have historically provided health care for those in need, often for persons who had no family. "From the second to the fifth century, the bishops' deacon cared for five specific groups: foundlings, orphans, the aged, pilgrims and the sick," writes Keenan. "Like the foundlings and the orphans, the aged had no family to assist them. Similarly the sick were without family and were more likely newcomers, transients, or pilgrims."[9]

The activity of the Church in health care, and the work of Catholic leaders in AIDS prevention in Nairobi are obviously works of mercy. Yet, they are so important for humanity in general because they serve a practical purpose—the sick need to be cared for just as the hungry need to be fed and the dead need to be buried. Since the very beginning of the Church, Catholics have been charged with the responsibility of discharging these corporeal works for those without family, thereby creating a family of faithful, united in the salvific message of Jesus Christ. As Fr. Keenan rightly states, "Since the moment Jesus first healed the sick, Christians have followed in his steps individually and collectively. With courage, compassion, wisdom, and imagination, the disciples of Christ continue in that long-practiced work of mercy."[10]

Reflecting on this long tradition of health care within Catholicism, priests and nuns in contemporary Nairobi consistently engage in works of mercy directed toward those living with HIV and AIDS, specifically through prevention efforts. And, what unites the family of Christians is not that they are motivated by some tangible reward, but rather they perform these works of mercy because of the practical need that exists in the society—just as Catholics have done since time immemorial. HIV and AIDS prevention motivated by mercy, then, represents an attractive comparative focus with Islamic notions of mercy.

Islamic Scripture and Mercy

"On the human plane, compassion—the capacity to feel and be with (*com*) the other in their suffering (*passio*)—expresses not just human sentiment but also spiritual presentiment," writes Islamic scholar Reza Shah-Kazemi. "Compassion arises first and foremost out of one's innate sense of the interconnected oneness of all human beings."[11] As a quintessential element of mercy, compassion informs Muslim efforts in prevention in Kenya's capital city particularly as compassion concerns the heart of the believer, which then reflects God's divine Mercy or *rahmah*. And, as indicated in the above quotation, there exists within Islam the central idea of the comprehensive interrelatedness and unity of all humanity.

In the words of Islam's most revered scripture, the Qur'ān, "Your creation and your upraising are as but as a single soul."[12] This unity of being is a central belief within Islam, which by further extension points to the unicity of God (Arabic, *tawhīd*). As a matter of interest, it is the concept of *rahmah*, the attribute of God, which also represents the tri-literal root of r-h-m originally referring to the womb and establishing the basic framework of two of God's divine Names, *Ar-Rahmān* and *Ar-Rahīm*, the Most Merciful and the Most Compassionate respectively. In its literal reference to God as the maternal source of all things, *rahmah* is singularly important in describing God's divine attributes, comprising "the qualities of compassion, mercy, forgiveness, loving goodness."[13]

Relevant to God's activity and identity, "the divine Names most clearly associated with mercy and compassion are given in a formula by which every significant act in Islam is consecrated, and with which every chapter of the Koran begins."[14] That mercy and compassion are so central to understanding God in Islam—as well as the relationship between man and God, and the relationship between man and fellow mankind—is remarkable as these two theological qualities manifest God's limitless love, even in the face of human folly since we are, in reality, the only ones who can be unmerciful.

In terms of actual scripture concerning mercy, perhaps the most often quoted *ayat* of the Qur'ān reads, "My mercy embraces all things."[15] This selection serves to set the parameters for the discussion of Islamic ideas regarding divine mercy since, by its very definition, God's mercy is infinite and "flows forth from the very nature of the Absolute."[16] Within Islam, God's mercy is manifest in all things at all times. God's infinite love, the impetus for creation, is evident in such Islamic scripture as, "I was a hidden

Treasure," says God, "and I loved to be known: hence I created creation/human beings (*al-khalq*), so that I might be known."[17] The very existence of mankind—including those Muslim leaders concerned with HIV and AIDS prevention—are contingent on God's love, mercy, and compassion without which the universe would cease to exist.

Thus, when we are confronted by the more formulaic equation found in the *Hadith* literature—with the divine saying, "My mercy takes precedence over my anger"—the result is unsurprisingly weighted in favor of God's limitless love and mercy. This *Hadith* obviously and candidly states that God is capable of anger. However, mercy and anger are not held in equilibrium. Rather, God's anger is brought about through human sin and anger itself is not an intrinsic attribute of God but rather one attributed to him through human agency. This is why Reza Shah-Kazemi notes, "Given the fact that among the divine Names one also finds 'the Almighty,' 'the Avenger,' and other names of divine rigor, it is of great significance that the formula of consecration [the *basmala*] contains a repetition of the theme of mercy." He continues, "one might have thought it more logical or balanced to include a name of rigor in this definitive consecration describing the essential nature of God in whose name one begins everything, and thus have something like: 'In the Name of God, the Compassionate, the Powerful.' "[18]

To reformulate the above assertion in different terms, mercy is a quintessential dimension of God's being motivated through infinite love whereas God's anger is a by-product of human sin—through both action and inaction. Divine anger, then, is "limited and relative, so the divine qualities elicited by relativity cannot be placed on the same level and those that flow forth from the very nature of the Absolute."[19] And, since God's mercy is absolute—encompassing everything and outweighing anger by scores—for us as humans it is comforting to know that God's love is directed toward each of us, though hopelessly incomprehensible for our human intellect to fathom. This is especially true when considering the relationship between human action and mercy. The Qur'ān explicitly states, "Whoso brings a good deed will have ten the like of it."[20] Yet, the Qur'ān continues, "whoso brings an evil deed shall only be recompensed the like of it; they shall not be wronged."[21] Instead of exacting vengeance on the evildoer, God assures an equilibrium for the evil deed—one for one—while rewarding the good deed tenfold. From this, it is evident that for God, good deeds far outweigh evil ones. This focus on human agency and responsibility is useful for understanding God's mercy. As the Qur'ān explicitly states regarding human activity, "Whatever good visits thee, it is of God; whatever wrong visits thee is of thyself."[22]

It would be a mistake at this point to think that any human action can have a direct effect of God. Instead, our shortcomings become evident when we fail to recognize that God's mercy surrounds us, everywhere and at all times. It is therefore the responsibility of the Muslim to recognize God's presence in the created world, in part by perfecting the soul through actions that reflect the divine Names of God. "Whenever God is described in terms of compassion and peace and love, it is always implied that the soul is being called upon to assimilate these qualities," Shah-Kazemi writes. "Those Names and qualities that characterize God must also characterize man—*mutatis mutandis*; what is true of God in absolute mode must be true of man in relative mode."[23] As man has been appointed the vicegerent over this world as *khalīfa*, God implores us to perform good deeds—even rewarding us unnecessarily when we do so—so that Muslims can continually strive to perfect their faith in religion (*islam*), action (*ihsan*), and faith (*iman*).[24] Even if we fall far from the ideal model of man—*al-insān al-kāmil*, represented in perfection by the Prophet Muhammad—we can be reassured that through God's mercy we can continue working toward that desired outcome.

Thus, even though humans have their shortcomings as faithful believers, God makes provisions for us to redeem ourselves, underscoring the interconnectedness of all humanity. For example, the "*Hadith* of the Questioning" presents a dialogue between God and a Muslim on the Day of Final Judgment:

> God says on the Day of the Rising: "O son of Adam, I was sick and you didn't visit Me." He said: "O my Lord, how could I visit You, and You are Lord of the worlds?!" God said: "Didn't you know that My servant so-and-so was sick, yet you didn't visit him? Or didn't you know that if you had visited him *you would have found Me with him*?" [Then God says:] "O son of Adam, did I not ask you for food, but you refused to feed Me?" He said: "O my Lord, how could I feed You, and You are Lord of the Worlds!?" God said: "Now didn't you know that my servant so-and-so asked you for food, but you didn't feed him? And didn't you know that if you had fed him *you would have found that with Me*?"[25] [Then God says:] "O son of Adam, I asked you for a drink, but you didn't give Me anything to drink." He said: "O my Lord, how could I give You a drink, and You are Lord of the Worlds!?" God said: "My servant so-and-so asked you for a drink, but you didn't give him any. But if you had given him a drink *you would have found that with Me*."[26]

The above is a very compelling predicament, since it presents starkly negative terms of human inadequacy—that the human being as a "son of Adam" did not visit the sick, nor did he give food to the hungry or offer drink to the thirsty.

Even in the Gospel of Matthew, all the sheep of the nations of the world are rewarded for their good deeds and only the goats who failed to do the corporeal acts of mercy are punished, thereby preventing them from entering the Kingdom of God. At least in the Christian equation, there is a relationship between reward and punishment whereas in the Islamic account, the human being is only reminded of when he failed to act in the ongoing process of human perfection. This, it would seem, hearkens back to the Islamic emphasis on human activity and how it can obfuscate man's ability to see the Real which exudes infinite mercy.

As a result, our failure to see God in the sick, the hungry, and the thirsty constitutes a systemic failure for all humans everywhere, reminding us that by nature, we are imperfect. The accompanying anger of God, then, "is nothing more but the extrinsic consequence of the lack of the soul's receptivity to the mercy that eternally radiated from the very nature of being."[27] It is not necessarily that the Muslim failed in being merciful to other humans, but rather the Muslim failed to recognize that everything is a reflection of God's divine mercy. Through being merciful, one is reflecting God's divine attribute through the mirror of their soul. And, as is the case in the Gospel of Matthew, when the faithful perform merciful deeds—visiting the sick, giving food to the hungry, providing drink to the thirsty—they are in essence acknowledging the interconnectedness of all things.

Even when we fail to act, as we see in this *Hadith*, God's bountiful mercy supersedes our shortcomings and reminds us that God's love is limitless. "Do not despair of God's mercy," the reassuring words of the Qur'ān read.[28] As this pertains to Muslim prevention efforts in Nairobi, it might be obvious that the "*Hadith* of the Questioning" may serve as a rallying call for religious officials working in the strategic aims of prevention and health care—particularly as this relates to HIV and AIDS in Kenya. That the *Hadith* is, again, formulated negatively is fascinating since many people living with the virus in Nairobi are oftentimes overlooked at best and at other times plainly ignored. Imams and sheikhs engaged in the discussion of prevention from an Islamic perspective are assured of doing God's own work by attending to the sick, since other members of the faithful community have failed in this area—just as God's interlocutor failed in his responsibilities toward his fellow man and, by extension, toward God.

Muslim leaders working in the field of health care and prevention are indeed performing works of divine mercy for those living with AIDS infection, while also helping to prevent future infection throughout the city. Through the course of performing these duties, these Muslim officials are participating in the continuing process of human perfection through works of mercy where others have failed in their responsibilities to the sick in their own communities.

Conclusion: Prevention and Mercy

While Islam and Catholicism maintain their own principled discourse toward those living with illness, there is an obvious overlap between the two faith traditions particularly in disease prevention and health care directed toward those individuals living with HIV. As scriptural accounts illuminate, the religiously faithful are called to attend both theologically and practically to those who are negatively affected by the AIDS epidemic in Nairobi. Indeed, mercy is at the heart of these efforts at disease prevention since, "whoso gives life to a soul, shall be as if he had given life to mankind altogether."[29]

For both Islam and Christianity, performing merciful deeds for those who have been marginalized, overlooked, or forgotten is to engage in the work of God whose unlimited mercy we reflect in our own actions directed toward members of our worldwide community. This is why the crossroads of religion and health care is so important for a comparison of the practical response to HIV and AIDS from both religious traditions. The very fact that religious representatives from within Islam and Christianity provide care for the physical dimension of the human being brings into focus mercy as functioning in the religious response to HIV and AIDS in Nairobi.

Catholics and Muslims reflect God's divine mercy through their own actions in disease prevention. Performing these merciful works for the human body, these leaders in Nairobi are creating a family of believers that transcends actual physical family bloodlines by visiting the sick, feeding the hungry, and giving drink to the thirsty. In caring for the whole human—that is physically and spiritually—Muslims and Catholics working in prevention and health care are doing God's work on earth by channeling God's infinite mercy, which encompasses all things.

EDUCATION AND HOSPITALITY

As a crisis, Sunni Muslim and African Catholic efforts in Kenya began with an improper understanding of how the human immunodeficiency virus was transmitted, its negative association with disordered sexuality, and the authority of the religious leaders within the community. Since the disease was associated at that early stage with people who had violated the established social order or with those who had acted immorally, education was difficult from a religious perspective since it often entailed a moral judgment on how the disease was contracted.

In terms of actual education in Kenya, both Islam and Christianity hold tremendous influence in changing how the population perceives the disease. More and more, priests and imams are speaking out about the virus from the pulpit, thus providing their congregations factually correct information on the nature of HIV—including its etiology and methods of effective prevention. This is perhaps one of the most important elements of education—that if the religious leaders are informed about the severity of the epidemic, then those same leaders can disseminate correct information about the virus within their own communities of faith.

This research identifies the common tradition of hospitality which is operative in the Muslim and Catholic efforts in the field of education. As arguably the largest group of non-governmental educators in Kenya, Islam and Catholicism throughout the past three decades have demonstrated an openness toward people living with HIV and AIDS infection, suspending moralistic judgment to witness, accompany, and stand in solidarity with them on their journey.

Therefore, education as a transformative power through a conceptual openness toward others to whom we may not be familiar is in itself a form of hospitality since clergy open themselves to learn from and attend to those living with infection while learning from leaders of other faith traditions. In turn, these leaders are teaching their congregations scientifically correct facts about disease transmission devoid of moral judgment, as the epidemic in Nairobi affects every member of the community regardless of infection status or religious self-identification. This section considers the theological roots of hospitality—first within Christian then Islamic scripture—to offer a comparative analysis of what it means to be hospitable, and how hospitality informs Catholic and Muslim ecumenical efforts in education.

Christian Scripture and Hospitality

Hospitality from within any of the three major monotheistic religions must necessarily begin with the example of Abraham. As the patriarch of the Abrahamic faiths—Judaism, Christianity, and Islam—Abraham is the quintessential example for how hospitality can be brought into concert with HIV and AIDS education in Nairobi. For Christians, Abraham holds a distinguished position in defining religious identity. A paragon of hospitality, the story of Abraham in the desert is well-known and serves as an example of opening our doors, families, and hearts to complete strangers for the benefit of our common humanity.

In the interest of time, a brief overview: Abraham and his wife Sarah are encamped in the desert when they were visited by three strangers. Not knowing he is being visited by God, Abraham rushes to the tent entrance to meet them, even though welcoming strangers in nomadic lands was always a potentially perilous act since one didn't know if the visitor was friend or foe. Yet, even though Abraham did not know the strangers, he shows them gracious hospitality—opening his house to them, washing their feet, and letting them rest. Not only that, but he even goes so far as to offer the men some of his prized goods:

> And Abraham hastened into the tent to Sarah, and said, "Make ready quickly three measures of choice flour, knead it, and make cakes." Abraham ran to the herd, and took a calf, tender and good, and gave it to the servant, who hastened

> to prepare it. Then he took curds and milk and the calf that he had prepared, and set it before them; and he stood by them under the tree while they ate.[30]

That Abraham and Sarah showed such hospitality and openness to complete strangers is remarkable, since we as humans are often wont to be gracious to people we do not know. This is, perhaps, the point—that Abraham and Sarah were able to see past these men as strangers in order to provide them with water to wash their feet, shade to rest, and the best food they had to offer. While there are definite parallels to the corporeal works of mercy examined in the preceding section—feeding the hungry and giving drink to the thirsty—it is interesting that both mercy and hospitality at their core are concerned with caring for the physical dimension of the human being.

In providing food and drink, the gracious host fills some sort of theological need as well. In the example of Abraham, welcoming the three strangers and acting as the generous host, he sets the standard justifiably high for the rest of us to achieve in our own lives, to demonstrate an openness to those who are different, those we don't know. And for his trouble, Abraham is blessed with a son to continue his bloodline even though he and Sarah are advanced in age and she questions whether they can have children in the first place. God then reassures her that, "Is anything too wonderful for the Lord? At the set time I will return to you, in due season, and Sarah shall have a son."[31]

Certainly a miraculous element to this story, Abraham and Sarah are rewarded and blessed for showing an openness—through hospitality—to the strangers. This is where hospitality as a conceptual openness to other humans can be identified in religious education programs in Nairobi. Since the early days of HIV in Kenya, Catholics have been instrumental in changing the way the general population view the disease. First, by educating themselves in the vocabulary of the virus, then educating others about the disease. In the process, Catholic leaders found themselves in a challenging though distinguished position—one which allowed priests and nuns to provide care by being open to other Catholics who were living with the virus. The hospitality as openness that many of these leaders have shown—not only in their own communities, but also to people from other faith traditions—reinforces the example of Abraham and Sarah in the desert with their three strangers.

Further, as is presented in the Epistle of Paul to the Hebrews, "Do not neglect to show hospitality to strangers, for by doing that some have entertained angels without knowing it."[32] The story of Abraham, as a story based in education, is itself instructive in terms of what is expected of the Christian community, particularly for people who are different from yourself. Interestingly, Catherine Cornille includes hospitality in her list of the basic parameters of interreligious dialogue. Though she presents hospitality as an openness or receptivity to the truth in other faith traditions, the example of

Abraham might be useful in spelling out why hospitality is so integral in the Christian conception of finding truth in strangers and how this relates to education.

"In the context of the dialogue between religions, the term "hospitality" is often used to designate the need to welcome the religious other in spite of religious difference," Cornille writes. "Here, however, we use it to imply an attitude of openness and receptivity to those very differences as a possible source of truth."[33] Whereas Abraham and Sarah did not know the strangers visiting their encampment, they still opened their tent and offered them the best hospitality they could muster. Where the biblical account did not state whether the strangers were of a different ethnicity or religion, by being open and receptive to them, the course of Abraham and Sarah's lives are changed forever through their hospitality to these strangers.

It is by affirming the inherent dignity and the common humanity of those that are different from ourselves that we can emulate the example of Sarah and Abraham. In this way, it is not merely offering hospitality to provide basic accommodations for the other—though this is one obvious element of caring for the human as a physical organism. Rather, it is through being receptive and open to the difference of the other that we ourselves can be changed—and often dramatically so—as with Abraham and Sarah through our experience of people who are strangers.

One central dimension of this understanding of hospitality focuses on education, what we can learn not only about the religious other but also what we can learn about ourselves through our encounter with the religious other. According to some who engage in interreligious dialogue, "the goal of dialogue is not to convince other religions of one's own superior truth or still less to convert individuals from one religion to the other, but to allow each participant to realize more fully the truth of their own religious tradition, and integrate that truth in their own lives."[34] The major focus of this approach to interreligious dialogue from a Christian perspective looks to some basic form of similarity between the various faith traditions dialoguing, while also being open to the possibility of learning from those very traditions.

Yet hospitality by its very nature is inclined to accommodate the differences of ritual, practice, and belief that exist between the religions of the world. After all, just as Abraham catered to those strangers who were unfamiliar—different—from himself and Sarah, Christian leaders working in education in Nairobi face the challenge of making sense of the basic truth of human experience. With an ethic of compassion based in the broad range of human experience of people living with HIV and AIDS in Kenya, there are similarities and differences in these personal experiences—as well as with interreligious interaction with people of different faiths in Nairobi:

> If hospitality toward truth in difference may lead to growth, it remains to be seen what types of religious change and growth one may reasonable envision through a progress of dialogue. It is of course impossible and against the very grain of dialogue to determine *a priori* the possible outcomes of any particular dialogue. The parameters of growth will always depend on the particular context and focus of any dialogue. But allowing for the necessary vigilance against what is irrelevant or opposed to one's own basic convictions, there are a number of avenues along which growth may exceed both the full abstraction and mutual ethical edification so often envisioned in interreligious dialogue.[35]

The above quotation identifies several important points to conclude this section on the Christian tradition of hospitality operating in the field of education in Kenya. First and foremost, given the breadth of aims and objectives of interreligious dialogue in general, it is first necessary to address the "particular context." In the case of this present study, the social context is the cosmopolitan city of Nairobi where Catholics—among other Christian denominations and persons of other faith traditions—interact daily. This exchange of religious ideas, practices, and beliefs has undoubtedly created a specific social milieu, one in which Catholic leaders serve and attend to the physical and religious needs of others through hospitality. From this open interaction with religious difference, clergy in Nairobi have streamlined their education efforts in the interest of efficiency to learn from those diverse and different.

Second, given the truth of the actual lived experience of those Catholics living with HIV and AIDS infection, there is both similarity and difference. Similarity, in that they are confessional Catholics living with the disease in a centralized geographic location. Difference, in that each of these individuals internalize and understand their own experience of living with the human immunodeficiency virus in different ways. The question then becomes one not of Divine Truth, but one of the truth of human experience and how the hospitality of those Catholic leaders working in AIDS education are helping to make sense of these similarities on a human level. Hospitality as receptiveness and openness to the truth—both human and divine—can lead Catholic clergy to a change in self-awareness, not only as religious beings but also as human beings.

Thus the example of Abraham comes full circle as the archetype of hospitality, which is largely applicable to the case of HIV and AIDS education, once more identifying its transformative power. A susceptibility to the experience of others, both from within our own religious tradition and from without, is an important dimension of intra- and interreligious education about AIDS in Kenya, from both the Catholic and the Muslim perspective.

Islamic Scripture and Hospitality

As the progenitor of Islam and a close friend of God (*hanīf* and *khalīl* in Arabic), Abraham is a major character in the Muslim imagination.[36] Not only did he break with the ways and beliefs of his native city—going against the polytheistic religion of his own father—he rebuilds the Ka'bah, the House of God and center of Islamic worship with his son Ishmael among other feats.[37] As a wholesome human, "Abraham is the model of human perfection, embodied *fitra* [the primordial state of belief and surrender to God], the father of monotheism, and the prophet who is understood as the closest in character traits to Muhammad."[38] It is, therefore, with some degree of attentiveness that we proceed to analyze the story of Abraham's hospitality in the revealed word of God to mankind, the Qur'ān.

Unlike the Judeo-Christian scriptural traditions which encapsulate the story of Abraham and Sarah in the desert to fifteen narrative lines in chapter 18 of the Book of Genesis—right before arguing with God over how many righteous individuals need inhabit the wicked cities of Sodom and Gomorrah to prevent God from razing them both—the comparative theologian can be emboldened by the fact that, in the Qur'ān, there are two different accounts of Abraham's hospitality, one in *Surah El-Hijr*, the other in *Surah Adh-Dharriyat*.

In the first account—*El-Hijr*—Abraham is visited by "guests." However, where in the Genesis account Abraham quickly made accommodation for his visitors, the Qur'ān states that Abraham proclaims, "Behold, we are afraid of you."[39] Fear at the sight of unexpected visitors was not an all too surprising reaction, as traders generally travelled in caravans throughout the Arabian Peninsula and one never knew if a solitary group of three riders was friendly or hostile.[40] However, God disabuses Abraham of his fear, telling him that they bring "good tidings of a cunning boy."[41]

In a departure from the Judeo-Christian account, it is not Sarah who questions whether she will be able to give birth to a child in her old age, but rather Abraham inquires, "What, do you give me good tidings, though old age has smitten me?"[42] Abraham, in this excerpt, sounds less like the paragon of hospitality and more like a doubting Thomas. The Lord, once again, is quick to ease Abraham's anxiety with the rejoinder, "We give thee good tidings of truth. Be not of those that despair," to which Abraham responds, "Who despairs of the mercy of his Lord, excepting those that are astray?"[43] While not explicitly about hospitality, Abraham does in the end acknowledge that, certainly, he does not despair of God's own limitless mercy and that he welcomes the good tidings of God in the form of his wise son.

It is intriguing that this Qur'ānic account departs from Abraham as a gracious host and instead points out his wholesome nature, which is interconnected with mercy. "Wholesomeness clearly derives from God's mercy," write Sachiko Murata and William Chittick, "since it results in nearness to God."[44] Indeed, this nearness to God also applies to being able to recognize God, which Abraham is clearly able to do in this version of the story. Relevant to this particular discussion is the relationship in the above narrative of mercy in hospitality. There are of course elements of mercy in hospitality—offering food, drink, and a place to rest for the weary stranger, even as God's own divine mercy is reflected in the hospitality shown to other humans.

This is evident in the second iteration of the story of Abraham in the desert found in *Surah Adh-Dharriyat*. In this selection, the entire tone is different since it is told from the perspective of God to the Prophet Muhammad and, in many ways, parallels the Genesis tradition. On being approached by three strangers who announce, "Peace," Abraham responds with "Peace! You are a people unknown to me."[45] Then, as in the biblical account, he offers his guests, though strangers, a "fatted calf" and asks them to eat. Yet, in keeping with the lines from *El-Hijr*, Abraham grew worrisome about his visitors: "Then he conceived a dread of them, They said, 'Be not afraid!' And they gave him good tidings of a cunning boy."[46]

On further analysis, the similarities between these two stories in the Qur'ān seem to outweigh the differences, though the message of each may be directed toward slightly different ends. In the latter account, Abraham's hospitality toward the uninvited guests is manifest as he offers them a greeting of peace and has a fatted calf cooked for them—no small trouble to him, to be sure. And yet, even having offered this gracious deed, he begins to fear the visitors. When juxtaposed with the Judeo-Christian tradition, this Islamic text paints Abraham in an all too human light since he questions his decision to open his home to the strangers and betrays the all too common human emotion of fear.

As the passage states, Abraham did not know the travellers, which might cause someone to turn the visitors away or act in an inhospitable manner. Even with this fear of the unknown, Abraham continues to be gracious and is rewarded for his actions. Conversely, in the former story, Abraham is presented as someone who is already afraid of the three unknown men—saying explicitly, "Behold, we are afraid of you."[47] It is then God who removes the fear from the patriarch's heart with good tidings, though Abraham is still skeptical. In each of these two narratives, there is an element of uncertainty intrinsic to the relationship between God and Abraham.

This emphasis on human nature adds a realism to the story of Abraham and the strangers, much more so than in the Jewish and Christian traditions. Particularly in pre-Islamic Arabia referred to in Arabic as the *Jāhīliyyah* or the days of Ignorance before the message of Islam, there was no certainty that a group of riders in the desert was offering good tidings. Rather, given the limited resources among the desert nomads, it was far more likely that these strangers were raiders resorting to the *ghazu* raid which was a common practice of the Bedouin, "as well as being a rough-and-ready means of redistributing resources in a land where there was simply not enough to go round."[48]

It would be understandable and a realistic human reaction for Abraham to sense fear at the arrival of his unannounced guests. Nevertheless, what is remarkable about the gracious acceptance of the visitors is that Abraham worked past his fears to offer the strange men food and a place to rest, the reason why Abraham is considered the model of hospitality. For even while Abraham resembles the perfect man (*al-insān al-kāmil*), to offer hospitality is to attend to the physical needs of other people—even if we are afraid. "Hospitality is the measure of the perfectability of man," which is a helpful point of departure from speaking scripturally about hospitality in order to show how this virtue—which "lies at the basis of the Islamic ethical system"—informs and motivates education efforts among Muslims in Nairobi.[49] As the history of the epidemic clearly demonstrates, the arrival of HIV in the early 1980s and its impact on the population of Kenya was nearly impossible to comprehend. Specifically in the area of education, imams and sheikhs could not educate the population because they simply did not then have the knowledge or vocabulary to do so. Further, since the disease carried moral judgment due to its association with sexuality, many Muslims were afraid of being educated about their own susceptibility to the virus for fear of actually knowing the truth about their status. The ensuing silence surrounding the early AIDS epidemic in Nairobi claimed untold scores of Kenyans as Islamic education on HIV failed these individuals.

However, in recent years, there has been a movement past this fear—fear of judgment, fear of talking about infection status, fear of discrimination and stigma—with Islamic leaders providing and implementing effective education programs in the local *madrasas* in Nairobi and outlying regions. In 2002, the Supreme Council of Kenyan Muslims, SUPKEM, created and instituted a comprehensive curriculum for teaching imams to be agents of change throughout Kenya concerning HIV and AIDS prevention and the destigmatization that was then supported by the government in all public schools.[50] Muslims, working in the field of education, can be considered as performing gracious acts of hospitality toward Muslims living with HIV infection in Nairobi.

At this point, it might be helpful to clarify precisely how hospitality relates to HIV and AIDS education in Nairobi, through the example of Abraham. As a model of being open to strangers—even in the face of his own fears—Abraham represents a compelling lens with which to view education as hospitality. As a basic human reaction and emotion, Abraham feared that which he did not know. It is in moving past his own fears of the unannounced visitors that he is finally able to offer true hospitality—opening his home and himself to the guest—in order to give and receive good tidings so that his life could be utterly transformed by God's presence. The receptivity to the unknown other, then, is the key to transformative hospitality.

> For Muslims, the concept of hospitality goes deeper into history than is commonly understood in the West. . . . For Arabs in particular, hospitality is an ancient concept. Pre-Islamic Arab civilization saw hospitality as a humanizing element that involves both the guest and host, creates trust between them, leads to an ennobling and transformative moment, and evokes a restorative energy crucial for the survival of the human race. Linked closely with honor and chivalry, hospitality was considered an act of unconditional surrender to the needs of others. Islam accepted this heritage at its very inception.[51]

The above quotation is particularly apt for this section for several reasons. First, as a matter of comparative enterprise, the above lines could equally be applied to Christianity with the quintessential example of Abraham. The patriarch surrenders to his visitors in all three monotheistic religious traditions, even though they are strangers. Second, the excerpt rightly identifies the inherent relationship between the guest and host, employing such language as "ennobling," "transformative," and "restorative" to describe the impact of hospitality. Third and final, the author makes the stark claim that hospitality is "crucial for the survival of the human race."

Similarly, sheikhs and imams in Kenya's capital city are faced with fear of the unknown with HIV and AIDS. However, like the figure of Abraham, these leaders are called to move past their own fears to be receptive to the lived experience of their fellow Muslims living with infection by radically reformulating their own conceptions and misconceptions about the epidemic. With duly altered minds and hearts, Muslim official in Nairobi can thus serve as agents of change within their own religious communities with their legitimacy as leaders to empower and transform the Muslim population through effective education.

Indeed, education at its very basis deals with being open and receptive to not only those foreign to us—like Abraham—but also relates to theories and concepts that we think we know. Through educational initiatives and curriculum development concerning the AIDS virus, Muslim leaders are changing preexisting notions of disease etiology and modes of transmission to transform public opinion based in a gracious openness and hospitality.

Conclusion: Education and Hospitality

Invariably, each of us will be the recipient of hospitality as well as the one who offers hospitality at some point during his or her life. As this pertains to education about HIV and AIDS in Nairobi in both the Catholic and Muslim traditions, teaching about certain topics—topics that may prove troublesome or uncomfortable such as HIV and AIDS—is a credit to the common good and can be a transformative and restorative moment between the religious leader as educator and members of the faithful community. Education, as with hospitality, in this light is indeed "considered an act of unconditional surrender to the needs of others."

As anyone engaged in education in general can attest, there is an innate openness and susceptibility necessary between both mentor and mentee that can lead to a transformation of both, just as with guest and host in hospitality. And thus, Muslim and Catholic officials working in the field of AIDS education in Kenya serve not only as facilitators in changing public knowledge about the epidemic, but they are also engaged in works of hospitality through affirming the lived human experience of those people living with HIV and AIDS infection.

DESTIGMATIZATION AND JUSTICE

One of the most difficult challenges for the Muslim and Catholic response to the HIV and AIDS epidemic in Kenya is that of destigmatization. Stated forthrightly, stigma is a problem because, even with advances in prevention and education, stigma mitigation involves changing popular perceptions that may or may not be true regarding the disease itself. The true hurdle in these efforts involves leaders from both traditions addressing the troublesome issues of disease transmission and its negative association with sexuality. Destigmatization efforts are therefore difficult to address from a very practical standpoint because people living with the virus must treat the disease as a medical condition. Yet, from a religious perspective, many Muslims and Catholics still morally judge those with HIV as people who have acted immorally or unethically.

The sting of stigma attaches itself to the identity of the person living with the disease and oftentimes is directed toward their family as well. Stigma represents an immaterial though powerful presence in the discourse surrounding AIDS, sexuality, and morality in Kenya's capital. In this formulation, Muslim and Catholic leaders must come together as agents of empowerment to change the hearts and minds of Kenyans concerning their views toward people living with HIV and AIDS infection.

Since stigmatization deals with how people with the virus are popularly viewed, priests and imams in Nairobi are working to radically reformulate how the disease is understood from a theological perspective. Stigma and discrimination by their very nature detract from how the infected person is welcomed and accepted by the religious community, and the theological virtue that motivates persons religious in this area can be identified as justice. As a matter of what is due to the individual as a proportion of the common good, social justice involves inherent human dignity, which must never be diminished due to stigma, discrimination, or HIV infection. Muslim and Catholic leaders working in destigmatization efforts can be emboldened by the virtue of justice since their work affirms the intrinsic dignity of the human person—in Catholicism as being created in the *imago dei* and in Islam as being a reflection of Gods divine attribute associated with justice (Arabic, *'adl*) and infinite love (Arabic, *rahma*).

It should, therefore, not matter whether someone is HIV positive or how they contracted the disease in the first place. In keeping a similar framework, this section offers an analysis of social justice from within the Catholic tradition, which is then applied to destigmatization efforts. The subsequent section offers an analysis of justice in Islam, which is then used to analyze the Muslim strategic objectives in stigma reduction. It then concludes with a comparison of both religious responses to HIV and AIDS stigma in Nairobi.

The Catholic Tradition of Justice

"Thus says the Lord," reads Jeremiah 9:23–24. "Do not let the wise boast in their wisdom, do not let the mighty boast in their might, do not let the wealthy boast in their wealth; but let those who boast boast in this, that they understand and know me, that I am the Lord; I act with steadfast love, justice, and righteousness in the earth, for in these things I delight, says the Lord."[52] As one of the cardinal virtues, justice perfects the will and inclines the individual to render what is due to each throughout the society. While there are, in fact, many different types of justice—distributive, retributive, and even justice in general—for the purposes of this project we will be looking at social justice as a major tradition in Catholic social teaching.

Catholic social teaching is the field of doctrine concerned with social justice or how to appreciate human life and affirm human dignity through individual and collective action. Justice, then, is intimately connected to the care of the human person which, in turn, is motivated by the divine directive that "You shall love your neighbour as yourself."[53] As a person, a free and intelligent being created in the image of God, man intrinsically has a basic human dignity that is far superior to the rest of the created world, his habitation, and his surroundings. "A single human soul is worth more than the whole universe of material goods," writes Jacques Maritain. "There is nothing higher than the immortal soul, save God. With respect to the eternal destiny of the soul, society exists for each person and is subordinated to it."[54]

As a matter of social justice, the human person is called to partake in the common good of society which "must flow back upon persons and that it includes, as its principle value, the access of persons to their liberty of expansion."[55] Justice, as it pertains to the common good, is the operating directive of Catholic destigmatization efforts in Kenya, insofar as justice is a balance of proportion. As St. Thomas Aquinas writes in *Summa Theologica*, "[j]ustice is the habit whereby one with a consistent and perpetual will renders to others what it due them."[56] As a matter of proportion, justice is chiefly concerned with balance that, in a community of free agents and individual actors, can easily become skewed.

From this, we can draft a model of social justice that holds the basic component of the community—the individual—as the necessary link to the social life of the community. This is an important point—the individual holds an undeniable and irrevocable innate worth as basic to human dignity—since as an equilibrium or balance, social justice affords a privileged place to the poor, the needy, and the sick within society as the starting point in the discussion of stigma. From this, Catholics can affirm the inherent dignity of all members of society, not only its Catholic contingent nor only those free of HIV and AIDS infection.

First, as a matter of social justice based in Catholic social teaching, church clergy serving in stigma mitigation must incorporate empathy, compassion, and care that the Christian community directs toward those members of society most in need. Second, as a matter of doing what is right, social justice entails basically creating a society within which the dignity of the human person is consistently maintained and observed. Based in scripture, the Book of Proverbs offers: "[w]hen justice is done, it is a joy to the righteous, but dismay to evildoers."[57] In this selection, the balance is drawn between the righteous who seek justice and the evildoers who seek injustice. This supposes a society within which all seek justice—and in the case of destigmatization, social justice—where the human person can flourish.

And yet, as St. Augustine notes in *Concerning the City of God against the Pagans*, human justice is ephemeral and the best that society can attain here in the created world is a basically well-ordered society, which itself is a pale reflection of God's own divine justice. On earth, we strive for social justice even as it is out of our collective reach. "I cannot refrain from speaking about the city of this world," writes Augustine, "a city which aims at domination, which holds nations in enslavement, but is itself dominated by that very lust of domination."[58] In principle, the plight of the suffering of the least well-off must be acknowledged as one of the motivating factors in the discussion of stigma mitigation efforts in Nairobi, based in the Catholic vocabulary of justice grounded in attention to the common good.

"Biblically and theologically grounded norms of justice, as the inclusion of all in the common good with a preferential option for the poor," writes the Catholic theologian Lisa Sowle Cahill on the interplay between theology and society, "should energize and renew a theological ethics of inclusion, participation, equality, and empowerment, especially for the least well-off."[59] Looking to the social justice voice of religion, Cahill argues that understanding social context is necessary to address the myriad theological and ethical questions facing contemporary religious and secular society, as we saw in the first chapter. Advancing the Catholic social ethic based in justice, the common participatory nature of religious experience lends itself to a model of justice as participation in the common good. Related to theology and context, both religious and secular influences are important in understanding just how justice is understood by a particular society, which is motivated by a commitment to social justice and the common good.

In the case of HIV and AIDS in Nairobi, approaching the discussion in terms of the participatory common good tradition of Catholic social teaching, by affirming the inherent dignity of those afflicted with the virus it is then possible to focus on the place of justice and how this justice touches everyone within society—specifically those most marginalized members. Understanding the human context—that is, its social, anthropological, indigenous, religious, and above all cultural influences—of any response to stigma is singularly important since this activity does not operate in the realm of theory, nor does it operate in isolation. Religious and lay leaders working in stigma mitigation must engage the present epidemic and view the disease and the effects of the disease in human terms, with human faces incorporating realistic human behavior. The Catholic community in Nairobi cannot consider itself immune from the negative impact of HIV and AIDS on their own congregations.

Subsequently, religion interacts with society, which interacts with culture—echoing Cahill's assertion that the Catholic Church cannot stand alone outside of the epidemic. Rather, Catholics must self-consciously consider how the language of social justice can present an opening for dialogue through the external threat of AIDS in their community. As was considered in the previous chapter, a pivotal aspect of the religious response to HIV and AIDS in Kenya involves those religious figures working in the field of destigmatization. Catholic leaders, therefore, can and indeed are bringing about the preferential and effective attention to the dignity, needs, and rights of people living with the virus in terms of social justice partly through biomedicine and partly through faith.

Indeed, one major ethical dilemma pertaining to the HIV and AIDS epidemic in Kenya is in many cases, it makes the most marginalized poor even poorer.[60] Even in light of government subsidies, the cost of anti-retroviral drugs remain prohibitively expensive for the poorest, notwithstanding that these drug therapy regimens must be taken with food to be effective. This vicious cycle acts to detract from the autonomy of those suffering from such a debilitating and socially stigmatized disease. Basically, this social reality is unjust.

In the later stages of the disease, men and women are so weak that they can no longer work, resulting in a loss of income which places stress of care on other family members. When viewed from the lens of social justice, HIV deprives the individual person of the ability to develop their full potential, thereby robbing them of their basic human dignity. Within Catholic social teaching, the dignity of the poor living with any form of illness must not be diminished because of suffering or sickness, and these vulnerable members of society must never be excluded from the common good of society.

In this way, the Catholic Church is called to participate actively in the religious response to HIV. By acknowledging the dual identity of AIDS as a medical condition that raises questions both of a physical and theological nature, based in social justice in the field of stigma mitigation, Catholic officials are called to move past the negative aspects of the epidemic to instead emphasize the salvific nature of the Church, living and operating not only within Kenya specifically, but throughout the world.

Returning to the distinction between crisis and *kairos*, in affirming the inherent dignity of people living with disease by challenging preconceived notions about AIDS transmission that give rise to stigma, there exists the historical paradigm shift from darkness to light that allows the Catholic Church to act as a sign and instrument of the compassionate and just God that redeems and fulfills humanity, even through this devastating epidemic. As a community of believers concerned with social justice, the Church defines and achieves its mission within the contextual society. Yet as a health-care provider, it additionally serves the physiological needs of the congregation through just deeds aimed at destigmatization.

The Islamic Tradition of Justice

"*Tawhid* [the principle of God's unicity] means that people have nothing positive that is strictly their own; on the contrary, all good is in God's hands," write Murata and Chittick. "If people experience good, they experience it on God's initiative through no merit of their own. If they do not experience good, that is simply what they deserve, since—apart from God's blessing and mercy—they are literally nothing. Hence the Koran pictures human pretensions to good as distortions of the way things are."[61] With this excerpt, the good that we as humans believe emanates from our just actions does not really belong to us at all. Instead, goodness is all God's, a central belief of *tawhīd*, which encompasses God's mercy and blessing. How then does this relate to justice?

> No one is hurt, however, by human pretensions, except those that make the pretension. Justice (*'adl*) is a divine attribute, defined as putting a thing in its proper place. The usual opposite of *'adl* is *'zulm* which in the Koranic context we translate as "wrongdoing." Wrongdoing is a human attribute, usually defined as putting something in the wrong place. The Koran repeatedly stigmatizes human wrongdoing. Interestingly, when it mentions those who are harmed by the wrongdoing, it almost always employs the word self (*nafs*). People cannot wrong God. A mosquito cannot sting the sun. But people can

> and do wrong themselves every time they put something in the wrong place. They distort their own natures, and they lead themselves astray.[62]

With this understanding of justice—which bears a striking similarity between Augustine's City of God and City of Man, we have a fascinating distinction dealing with human agency. That is, whereas *'adl* as justice is one of God's divine attributes, its converse of *zulm* as wrongdoing is strictly associated as the result of human action or inaction. Wrongdoing therefore is a human attribute, the result of placing things in the wrong place, attributing partners to God (Arabic, *shirk*), or even failing to recognize the divine reflection of God's *tawhīd* in other humans. Humans who act unjustly are not harming God by any means—to do so would be impossible. Instead, humans only serve to harm themselves through performing wrong or unjust acts. As the Qur'ān asserts, "And We wronged them not, but they wronged themselves; their gods availed them not that they called upon, apart from God, anything, when the command of thy Lord came; and they increased them not, save in destruction."[63]

As this quotation relates to stigma mitigation in Nairobi, Muslim leaders working with people infected with HIV must be aware of the inherent injustice of discrimination as well as the injustice of the very structures that allow the disease to continue to spread. Because of this, stigma has both theological and practical implications since, "God's call to all of humanity to be maintainers of justice is an imperative no only to secure a just order on earth, but also most importantly, to ensure that all humans are able to worship only God—to be only His servants—and to be free from any persons, structures, or circumstances that force an individual to be in need of anything other than God."[64]

This observation candidly address the distinction between *'adl* and *zulm*, since to stigmatize against another member of the faithful Muslim community on the grounds of HIV infection status is to act unjustly, providing a misplaced and misinformed understanding of the disease, confusing the very foundation that the created world is set upon. With the story of the creation of Adam, the Qur'ān offers a glimpse into how the world was meant to be naturally ordered. God, in all of God's infinite power and wisdom, created Adam to be God's vicegerent (Arabic, *khalīfa*) and shared with Adam the knowledge of the names of everything in creation. As the Qur'ān recounts, "And He taught Adam the names, all of them," and "Adam, tell them their names."[65] Thus, in Adam's position as vicegerent over the earth, all of creation is subjugated to the fully human being, since "A vicegerent is someone who is given the authority and the means to lead in someone else's stead. When God taught Adam the names, he gave him a share of his own ruling power."[66]

As a representative of God on earth, humans have the power—based in God's own power—to change their relationship with the world around them both for the better or the worse. This is especially true governing the relationship between humans themselves. Discrimination and stigma, then, are particularly troublesome social developments since they are negative claims against fellow vicegerents, inasmuch as "[t]he human being was also created in God's form, embracing all of God's attributes. The difference between the whole universe and the human being is that the signs are infinitely dispersed in the universe, while they are concentrated into a single, intense focus in each individual."[67]

The human soul thus acts as a mirror of these divine attributes, which in effect gives the individual Muslim the freedom and responsibility to negotiate their relationship with the world around them. To stigmatize or discriminate against a fellow human being is to deny this very basic reflection of God's divine nature:

> The concentration of the attributes within human beings makes people God's vicegerents, that is, creatures who can perform the same functions as God, with all due respect to *tanzih* [God's incomparability]. Human beings manifest all God's attributes, but in a weakened and dim manner, demanded by the fact that, although they are similar to God in respect of having been created in his form, they are different in respect to spatial and temporal limitations. God remains infinitely beyond any human being.[68]

As this concept relates to stigma mitigation in Nairobi, Islam promotes a privileged place for those ignored or overlooked by the rest of society—the poor, orphans, widows, and the elderly. This is precisely because, as Murata and Chittick rightly identify—they are all manifestations of God's divine love. Additionally, these members of Islamic society are quintessential components of the *'ummah*, a term denoting the broadest sense of the Muslim community throughout the world. Indeed, many of the first converts to Islam were among the most marginal elements of pre-Islamic Arabian society, and the unifying message of Islam served to critique and perfect the traditions that had come before.[69]

As Islamic theologian Abdulaziz Sachedina rightly states, "God's abstract justice has found concrete expressions in the health care provided to the destitute and downtrodden."[70] However, questions remain as to how this justice is understood in specifically Muslim societies, as well as how this justice can and should be applied to all the members of the community. Understanding the human context within which justice operates is equally as important to understanding how justice is distributed. When applied to the Muslim initiatives in stigma mitigation for those living with the virus, the individual—as *khalīfa*—is supremely important, since the universe has been subjugated to each of us, including as well the perpetrator of stigma.

Human wrongdoing, *zulm*, is then the cause of this negatively or misplaced, disordered reality and is to blame for stigma and stigmatization. Further, *zulm* is injustice since it seeks to ignore the actual experience of people living with disease who themselves reflect God's essence. To overlook or ignore those sick in our own societies is to deny the omnipresence and omnipotence of God who implores us to care for the needy in our own lives. "At the most basic level, the Qur'an speaks to this in the necessity to support the weakest members of society," writes Buysse. "The Qur'an places the imperative on humans to support all weak members of society unconditionally, regardless of religious affiliation or 'moral behavior.' "[71]

This last point—that Muslims should strive in justice to provide basic support to the needy in society regardless of moral behavior or confessional identity—identifies the central issue of stigma, that the moral judgmentalism has made providing recourse to all living with infection difficult:

> It is clear that an effective response to AIDS has been hindered in part by the stigma and relative powerlessness of many of its victims: sex workers, intravenous drug users, prisoners, migrant workers, gay and bisexual men, women, and people of color. . . . The Qur'an, however, insists that its listeners maintain justice in spite of passions, to "follow not the lusts, lest you may avoid injustice." (4:135)[72]

Especially as this relates to the Muslim population in Nairobi confronting the very real threat of HIV and AIDS, the idea that God is with the sick is central to any approach to stigma mitigation and reduction, particularly in terms of interreligious dialogue. The faithful, both Catholic and Muslim, are called to offer care as justice for the most marginalized members of society—to visit the sick, feed the hungry, and give drink to the thirsty.

This understanding of justice looking to the interconnectedness of all humanity goes back to the point that as God's appointed vicegerents here on earth, we are continually redefining our relationship with the created world as well as with our fellow humans. "God desires to make clear to you, and to guide you in the institutions of those before you, and to turn toward you; God is All-knowing, All-wise," the Qur'ān advises. "God desires to turn toward you, but those who follow their lusts desire you to swerve away mightily. God desires to lighten things for you, for man was created a weakling."[73] Such a Qur'ānic injunction is instrumental not only for the Muslims of Kenya but is largely applicable to the rest of humanity. People living with AIDS are friends, brothers, sisters, mothers, and fathers; they are interrelated to us, not only in terms of genealogy but also in terms of being human beings, Christian and Muslim alike.[74]

Our ability to pass moral judgment against someone living with infection in the form of stigma and discrimination is an injustice, for it goes against the very roots of our religious traditions. As the Qur'ān explicitly advises, our passions must not lead us to be unjust. Thus, we are forced to reassess our understanding of the created world in light of our ability to do wrong and misplace things—such as to overlook the central importance of all God's vicegerents including notably those living with AIDS infection. Through Muslim and Catholic strategic efforts in destigmatization, leaders in Nairobi strive to create a just society which serves to insure that people living with HIV and AIDS are cared for as reflections of God's own divine majesty.

Conclusion: Stigma and Justice

Though the above quotation was posed by the South African Islamic theologian Farid Esack, it is equally applicable to Catholicism since the epidemic—not only in Kenya but worldwide—affects how people living with HIV and AIDS are treated, in general, by society. The stigma and discrimination directed toward those negatively affected by the disease, their families and friends, thus, serves to undermine the inherent worth of the human person, which is invaluable.

Whether this worth is understood as being created in the *imago dei* such as in the Catholic tradition, or as the human reflection of God's own divine attributes as with Islam, perceiving them negatively or preventing them from partaking in the common good of society is a form of injustice. Catholic and Muslims officials in Nairobi are thus charged with a difficult yet worthy task—to affirm the inherent dignity of those living with infection through their efforts in destigmatization. And, as the above quotation affirms, the AIDS crisis illuminates the general breakdown of the basic structures of society that themselves aim to allow the human person to develop themselves and achieve their full human potential. Stigma, as Esack rightly states, is one of the tragic symptoms of the injustice of the world. Interreligiously, Muslim and Catholic leaders working in the area of stigma mitigation are addressing the injustice of discrimination directed toward people living with HIV and AIDS infection in Nairobi.

CONCLUSION

Since much of this chapter has dealt with scripture, this conclusion began with a selection from the Qur'ān in which God distinguishes between the true believers by physically testing their human bodies. When struck with a wound, the believer is comforted by the divine sanction that, "such days we deal out in turn among men, and that God may know who are believers, and blot out the unbelievers." The scripture continues interrogatively, "Or did you suppose you should enter Paradise without God knowing who of you have struggled and who are patient?"[75] In this account, the believer is called to be patient in the face of the struggles one encounters in life, including disease and suffering.

In demonstrating perseverance, believers are purified so that they can more fully understand God's divine presence in their own lives. When framed in scriptural terms, Islamic activity in the fields of prevention, education, and destigmatization serves to afford both religious leaders and lay practitioners with a new understanding of the etiology of diseases such as AIDS. This is also true of Catholic initiatives in the three areas considered in this chapter. By giving people open forums and the scriptural and theological vocabulary to intelligently speak about HIV and AIDS, Muslim and Catholic leaders throughout Kenya are comprehensively addressing the real threat of the virus within their own communities using the voice of mercy, hospitality, and social justice.

Indeed, each of these three theological traditions and virtues are operative in Catholic and Muslim strategic aims in the lived response to HIV and AIDS in Nairobi. It is only through addressing and understanding social context that we can even begin to fathom the depth and importance of the responses of these religious communities in Kenya to prevention, education, and destigmatization. "There is in every culture an admixture of the ethnocentric, bound to a particular geography, history, language, and ethnic strain; and the universal, which is common to all humans as humans," writes Abdulaziz Sachedina.[76]

The virtues of mercy, hospitality, and justice as explored in this chapter are of this latter, universal category since all three relate to humans as humans. With this in mind, religious leaders are called to work alongside other religious groups in addressing and alleviating the pain of those afflicted with such diseases as HIV and AIDS, both practically and spiritually. After all, Catholic ethicist Lisa Sowle Cahill stresses that religious institutions must assume a social engagement—not just a theory—but an actual engagement within the community within which ethical decisions are made. As this relates to prevention, education, and destigmatization and their corresponding theological virtues, we return again to the historical dimension of the epidemic in Nairobi, as a movement from crisis to *kairos*. While the crisis of HIV and AIDS is the perfect time for God's decisive action, it also underscores the call for a new strategy of Catholic and Muslim pastoral and medical care for those living with infection by addressing the social context of the epidemic in Kenya and responding appropriately to those in need.

As has been examined in this chapter, this new strategy is not static but has evolved over time. In the area of prevention, the mercy Muslim and Catholic officials direct toward those living with AIDS as a medical condition can be seen in the deeper human directive to visit the sick and provide care to the physical human being. In education, Muslims and Catholics open their doors, hearts, and minds to the lived experience of people living with the virus. And in stigma mitigation, these leaders are reassured in their efforts through the call for social justice and the common good tradition, from which those living with HIV and AIDS must never be excluded.

NOTES

1. The quotation at the beginning of this chapter comes from the Holy Bible, James 2:13. The quotation itself begins, "For judgment will be without mercy to anyone who has shown no mercy."
2. Bible, Matt. 25:31–40.
3. James F. Keenan, SJ, *The Works of Mercy: The Heart of Catholicism* (Lanham, MD: Rowand and Littlefield Publishers, 2007), 3.
4. Ibid., 4.
5. Bible, Matt. 25:40.
6. Rodney Stark, *The Rise of Christianity: How the Obscure, Marginal Jesus Movement Became the Dominant Religious Force in the Western World in a Few Centuries* (San Francisco: Harper San Francisco, 1997), 112–13.
7. Bible, 1 Corinthians 1:2.
8. Keenan, *The Works of Mercy*, 4.
9. Ibid., 46. He continues, "The deacons' care for pilgrims and the sick was a particularly onerous duty in pilgrimage centers. These centers of hospitality would eventually appropriately be called "hospitals."'
10. Ibid., 50.
11. Reza Shah-Kazemi, *My Mercy Encompasses All Things: The Koran's Teaching on Compassion, Peace, and Love* (Berkeley, CA: Counterpoint, 2007), 3.
12. Translations of the Qur'ān are from *The Koran Interpreted: A Translation*, trans. A. J. Arberry (New York: Touchstone, 1996). Qur'ān, 31:28.
13. Shah-Kazemi, *My Mercy Encompasses All Things*, 5.
14. Ibid.
15. Qur'ān, 7:156.
16. Shah-Kazemi, *My Mercy Encompasses All Things*, 7.
17. James W. Morris, *Openings: From the Qur'an to the Islamic Humanities* (Personal Manuscript, 2010), 68.
18. Shah-Kazemi, *My Mercy Encompasses All Things*, 5–6.
19. Ibid., 7.
20. Qur'ān, 6:160.
21. Ibid.
22. Ibid., 4:79.
23. Shah-Kazemi, *My Mercy Encompasses All Things*, 11.
24. Sachiko Murata and William Chittick, *The Vision of Islam* (St. Paul, MN: Paragon House, 1994), xxxii.
25. As James Morris notes, "This literal translation seems to accord with the intentional reference to the "eschatological" context here—in which the souls of those being judged are themselves understood to be suffering from the spiritual "hunger" and "thirst" often mentioned in those contexts in the Qur'an." Morris, *Openings*, 438.
26. Ibid., 438.
27. Shah-Kazemi, *My Mercy Encompasses All Things*, 10.
28. Qur'ān, 39:53.
29. Qur'ān, 5:32.
30. Bible, Gen. 18:6–8.
31. Ibid., 18:14.
32. Ibid., Heb. 13.2.
33. Catherine Cornille, *The Im-Possibility of Interreligious Dialogue* (New York: The Crossroads Publishing Company, 2008), 177.

34. Ibid., 187.
35. Ibid., 205.
36. Qur'ān, 4:125.
37. For Abraham's father, see Qur'ān, 6:47; 19:41–50. For rebuilding the Ka'bah, see Qur'ān, 2:125–127.
38. Murata and Chittick, *The Vision of Islam*, 290.
39. Qur'ān, 15:52.
40. Karen Armstrong, *Muhammad: A Biography of the Prophet* (San Francisco: Harper San Francisco, 1993), 58–60.
41. Qur'ān, 15:53.
42. Qur'ān, 15:54.
43. Qur'ān, 15:56.
44. Murata and Chittick, *The Vision of Islam*, 290
45. Qur'ān, 51:25.
46. Qur'ān, 51:28.
47. Qur'ān, 15:52.
48. Karen Armstrong, *Islam: A Short History* (New York: Random House, Inc., 2000), 19.
49. Snjezana Akpinar, "Two Responses to 'Interreligious Dialogue and Spiritual Hospitality': Hospitality in Islam," in *Religion East and West* 7 (2007), 24.
50. Some of the major challenges underscoring a Muslim bioethical response to HIV/AIDS came from a general misunderstanding of the roots of the pandemic and incorrect information on how the disease is transmitted. Educating the population attends to both the physical and spiritual nature of Muslims by addressing the concerns that underlie the perceived stigma associated with HIV/AIDS. Charles Nzioka, Allan Korongo, and Roseanne Njiru, *HIV and AIDS in Kenyan Teacher Colleges: Mitigating the Impact* (Paris: International Institute for Educational Planning, 2007), 24.
51. Akpinar, "Two Responses to 'Interreligious Dialogue and Spiritual Hospitality': Hospitality in Islam," 23.
52. Bible, Jeremiah 9:23–24.
53. Bible, Mark 12:31
54. Jacques Maritain, *The Person and the Common Good*, 6.
55. Ibid., 55.
56. Thomas Aquinas, *Summa Theologica*, trans. Fathers of the English Dominican Province (Brewster, MA: Christian Classics, 1981), II-II, q. 58, a. 1.
57. Bible, Proverbs 21:15.
58. Augustine of Hippo. *The City of God,* trans. Marcus Dods DD (New York: The Modern Library), I. i.
59. Lisa Sowle Cahill, *Theological Bioethics: Participation, Justice, and Change* (Washington, DC: Georgetown University Press, 2005), 16.
60. See Kelly, *HIV and AIDS*, 113–16.
61. Murata and Chittick, *The Vision of Islam*, 113.
62. Ibid.
63. Qur'ān, 11:101.
64. Caitlin Yoshiko Buysse, "The Qur'an, Poverty, and AIDS" in *Islam and AIDS*, 169.
65. Qur'ān, 2:31. The names here being understood as all of the divine "names" or "attributes."
66. Murata and Chittick, *The Vision of Islam*, 122.
67. Ibid., 123.
68. Ibid.
69. al-Tabriz, *Mishkat al-Masabih*, Vol. 1. One *Hadith* reads, "Men are of different origins just as gold and silver are; the best among them in the pre-Islamic period are the best among them in Islam when they are versed in the religion," 50. Another reads, "Among my people there are four characteristics belonging to the pre-Islamic period which they do not abandon: boasting of high rank, reviling other people's genealogies, seeking rain by the stars, and wailing," 361. Further, the Qur'ān, 17:81–82 reads, "The truth has come, and falsehood has vanished away; surely falsehood is ever certain to vanish."

70. Abdulaziz Sachedina, *Islamic Biomedical Ethics: Principles and Applications* (New York: Oxford University Press, 2009), 13.

71. Buysse, "The Qur'an, Poverty, and AIDS," 180.

72. Ibid., 180–81.

73. Qur'ān, 4:27–28.

74. Writes South African Muslim scholar, Farid Esak, "The resources for a global health care system that puts the human needs first do exist today. The struggle for justice is a struggle to make resources available to all. A theology of compassion, responsibility, and justice must thus make the connection between compassion on the one hand, and power or, more appropriately, the lack of it, on the other. AIDS (or any other disease) is not an isolated entity; the pandemic is just as much about a crisis and collapse of all social security structures in society as it is about a crisis and collapse of the immune system of the body. In many ways, the actual disease is one tragic symptom of the major injustices of the world, particularly the growing gap between the rich and the poor. The context of our struggle to bring dignity to those living with this condition is part of a larger one where the obscured connections between disease and socioeconomic conditions and processes are interrogated." Farid Esack, "Introduction," in *Islam and AIDS*, 6–7.

75. Qur'ān, 3:140–42.

76. Sachedina, *Islamic Biomedical Ethics*, 249.

Chapter Four

"Let anyone among you who is without sin be the first to throw a stone at her"

Lingering Questions of Sexuality and Areas of Unaddressed Concern

INTRODUCTION AND PLAN FOR THE CHAPTER

This chapter addresses some further practical implications arising from the broader issues raised in the preceding chapter.[1] The content of my research has relied heavily on the actual voices of Muslim and Catholic leaders interviewed in Kenya's capital. As a document that includes a historical record—seeking to offer a snapshot of intra- and interreligious efforts in HIV and AIDS prevention, education, and destigmatization—I began by striving to listen to those leaders using their own words to explain the religious as well as the sociocultural milieu which they largely inherited from previous generations of religious leaders.

These accounts provide a rare glimpse into the lives of both Muslim and Catholic officials trying to make sense of their faith in the face of inadequate health care, faulty education, and the enormous stigma directed toward those living with the virus throughout Kenya. The AIDS epidemic in this East African country is not the root cause of these wider developments and behaviors, but in many ways rather is a tragic symptom of them. As Lisa Cahill expertly attests, "AIDS requires that we address global structures of wealth and poverty, as well as market-based medicine and research, and cross-cultural norms for sex and gender, especially those that result in the oppression (and death) of women."[2]

Here, Cahill provides a realistic assessment of the challenge that religious officials face in responding to HIV and AIDS. What is needed then is an interdisciplinary approach that incorporates not only the work of medical professionals but also governmental officials and religious leaders working alongside each other in the promotion of the common good of society for all those living with illness. The prospect is no doubt daunting. "Social inequalities and conflicts between personal dignity and the common good will never be entirely eradicated," concludes Cahill.[3] And yet, in this project, Muslim and Catholic leaders in Nairobi are coming together to attend and serve people living with AIDS infection motivated by the theological traditions of mercy, hospitality, and justice.

This chapter proceeds as follows. Adapting the framework employed in the third and fourth chapters, it relies heavily on the firsthand accounts of interviews with Catholic and Muslim religious officials to discern one major area of common concern that was not highlighted as such in the preceding chapters. Related to both Islam and Christianity as lived traditions, sexuality is a topic many leaders and clergy—as well as their followers—find problematic, specifically in three areas: sexual relations, gender roles, and condom use.[4] The first half of the chapter presents Catholic views on those three areas related to sexuality using the interview material to examine the breadth of opinion on each topic. The second half of the chapter offers Islamic views related to sexual intercourse, gender roles, and condom use as this pertains to the HIV and AIDS epidemic in Nairobi.

CHRISTIANITY, ISLAM, AND SEXUALITY

Arguably one of the largest areas of consideration that has been explicitly and tangentially touched upon throughout this project is the problematic topic of sexuality. As is perhaps clear from the discussion of stigmatization, HIV has a long and problematic association with sexuality. In the words of Cahill, "When AIDS first came to the attention of Catholic moral theology, its analysis was closely connected to the morality of personal sexual behavior. Specifically, first-world moral theologians and Church teachers perceived AIDS as originating in sexual sin, especially homosexuality (and IV drug use)."[5] This foregone conclusion, that AIDS was somehow allied with sexual deviancy, gave rise to the belief that the remedy for AIDS was a stricter observance of sexual morality—specifically from a religious lens.

Within both the Catholic and Muslim communities in Nairobi, it has historically proven difficult to break through this negative view that people who contracted the disease had done so through some sort of taboo or violation of a social sexual norm, encouraged by popular opinion and religious views about the virus. For this reason, speaking about sexuality from a religious perspective has been a rather troublesome issue, most often met with silence. This section offers a comparative analysis of Muslim and Catholic views on sexual issues related to HIV and AIDS. Analyzing interview data collected during fieldwork, this section provides a unique perspective from leaders of both religions, as their responses provide a useful glimpse into how they understand the impact of HIV and AIDS in Nairobi and how they see themselves as official representatives of their religion.

Catholics Speaking about Sexual Intercourse

Both culturally and religiously, sexuality is a very difficult topic to broach with any interlocutor because of its intimate nature. In both religions, those not married are expected to abstain from sexual intercourse, while married persons are expected to remain faithful to their spouse. Any violation of this social order is met with moral judgmentalism—as seen in previous chapters—which can lead to stigma and discrimination. HIV serves to problematize the situation because of its myriad modes of transmission. Yet, sexuality remains a major area of focus in the discussion surrounding HIV and AIDS infection. In the words of one prominent Catholic educator, "sexuality is still a thorny—another thorny area."[6]

Because of its negative association with disordered sexual relations—homosexuality, infidelity, premarital sex—Catholic efforts in responding to the disease have been historically hampered by the silence and stigma regarding these private sexual acts. Even the institutionalization of a preferred Catholic social order has long been promoted in the ABC approach to HIV prevention and education. In this approach taught in most schools in Nairobi and promoted by many Catholic relief organizations, "A" stands for abstinence, "B" reminds students to be faithful, and "C" refers to using a condom with multiple sexual partners.

Nevertheless, the ABC's of AIDS prevention places emphasis on sexual intercourse as the only mode of disease transmission and does not acknowledge other channels of HIV infection, as Donald Messer notes, including "D for Drugs" and "E for Education."[7] Rather, there is a distinct focus on sexual relations, disproportionately says one Catholic nun. "Well first and foremost I say, throughout the world—the Catholic response, the emphasis on sexuality is disproportionate."[8] Keeping in line with the above discussion, this "disproportionate" emphasis on sexuality comes down to fundamental Catholic teaching that the unmarried must abstain from sexual acts and the married must stay faithful to their partners. "So consequently, extramarital sex or any acting out sexually—except within the context of marriage—is seen by the Church as incorrect," the sister continued. "And that emphasis is very strong in the whole presentation of the Christian faith in the Catholic context."[9]

With this framework based in Catholic teaching, there is the expectation that people will not have sexual intercourse outside the institution of marriage—but it doesn't address those people who have sex outside of marriage. With this rigid dichotomy, there is little room for human error—whether inadvertent or intentional. Surely the Catholic tradition teaches forgiveness for those who make mistakes. Yet, HIV serves to problematize the situation as a pathogen of both the society and the Catholic religion. "So because HIV is more heterosexually related here in Kenya than in the US, for example, where it is—it has been homosexually related," the nun stated.[10] Thus, the distinction between homosexual and heterosexual relations highlights an emphasis that disordered sexual acts are to blame for the continued spread of AIDS.

Of particular interest is the practical experience of people living with the disease and how they are viewed, treated, and accepted by the religious community. Even though it is a medical condition, from a popular perspective there remains the incorrect assumption that the disease is transmitted only through immoral sexual behavior which leads to condemnation. The nun concluded, "that would be my big faulting with the Catholic Church, is that because of the imbalance of sexuality, it has the effect for persons who have HIV of having a double condemnation."[11] The recurring theme of condemnation for this Catholic aid worker is twofold. On the one hand, the individual living with AIDS is condemned by the Church as someone who has acted in a morally disordered manner. On the other hand, they are physiologically condemned to live with the disease irrespective of how it was actually contracted.

Having one's basic human identity contingent on HIV status is, by its very nature, a systematic injustice—not only of secular society but also by persons religious. That this condemnation is directed toward their physical bodies as well as how they are viewed by other Catholics is worth noting since negative attitudes about AIDS must be addressed both practically and theologically so that people living with infection can be supported by the religious community with their inherent dignity affirmed. After all, the purpose of Catholic social teaching is to promote social justice.

Yet, Catholic education concerning AIDS and sexuality has let down many of those living with the disease in Nairobi. Within the field of education, one of the major challenges facing Catholic leaders in Nairobi lies in providing effective education to all Kenyans, not just Catholics. "So homosexuality is seen now as you know constitutes objectively disordered. Objectively disordered. And so all the [Church] teaching stems from that moral judgment. And so that's skewed as well," the nun concluded.[12] This "skewed" teaching on sexuality from the Church's perspective creates somewhat of a no-win situation. Either there is a disproportionate emphasis on disordered sexuality—as represented by the ABC's of AIDS prevention—or there is the skewed imbalance in Catholic education when teaching about sexuality, which is contested by certain dissident Catholic educators.

This distinction only addresses some of the issues pertaining to education. Indeed, there are several other factors leading to the negative association of AIDS with potentially incorrect notions of sexual intercourse. For example, there is also a connection between sexuality, poverty, and culture. "Looking at Kenya, I would say partially it could be poverty in some areas," replied one Catholic educator on the factors leading to AIDS infection. "That vicious cycle of poverty, where people don't see an outlet to it."[13] Hinting at the prospect of transactional sex for many women and men who have little other recourse, poverty is a major factor leading to the continued spread of AIDS throughout Nairobi.

Because of this negative association, HIV continues to be a topic that many people do not feel comfortable discussing openly. "I think issues surrounding sexuality—the silence that surrounds it," the official surmised. "People are not very open around issues of sexuality, and sometimes they don't seek help when they should. They're not able to freely discuss why it's going on."[14] Silence, shame, and stigma continue to be salient elements of the AIDS epidemic in Kenya, despite the noble efforts of Catholic leaders who work every day to combat these negative trends. Within the Catholic purview, sexuality and sexual intercourse continues to be an area of tension with its incommensurate emphasis in religious education, which is then aggravated by poverty. The HIV and AIDS crisis in Nairobi continues to be a challenge despite the advances already made in prevention, education, and destigmatization. This is also true of gender roles in Kenya, to which the present analysis now turns.

Catholics Speaking about Gender Roles

Another troublesome issue regarding sexuality is preconceived gender roles in contemporary Nairobi. According to social role theory, "men and women are expected to participate in activities that are in accordance with their culturally defined gender roles."[15] This division goes to the very self-identification of the individual, including which positions they hold, both publically and privately, how they are perceived in society, and even dictates which clothes they are expected to wear. When applied to the AIDS epidemic, the expectation of gender roles can even affect the division of labor for treating people living with the virus.

When asked who is addressing the practical needs of those negatively affected by the epidemic in Nairobi, one Jesuit priest candidly remarked, "Mostly sisters. This would be women in religious communities, and you will see that across the region of Eastern Africa. They are very, basically at the forefront of the response. And I would say they have been also the most effective in terms of their outreach to people in local communities, in terms of their care programs I think they have been the most effective."[16] Such statements are striking, particularly as the Catholic Church has a male-only hierarchy with priests and bishops making statements about HIV and AIDS that, in some cases, might be factually incorrect about disease etiology or modes of transmission. He further stated:

> I think that's a problem. In terms of how our priests are involved, I would say in terms of speaking about it, trying to inform the conscience of their communities. But not necessarily direct involvement like the religious women—communities of religious women—are involved in this. Again there are exceptions, I'm not saying that as a blanket statement. There are exceptions.[17]

This distinction between the sexes, especially with the Catholic hierarchy, is interesting particularly in the grassroots activism and the pastoral response affirming their dignity and giving witness to their experience.

The ministry of religious women fills the necessary gaps in the previously discussed strategic areas of prevention, education, and destigmatization. As a lived religious response, the nuns in Nairobi serve a very practical purpose of direct involvement in the community. The priest's observation about women religious highlights a fascinating distinction between the physical and the theological dimensions of the AIDS epidemic in Kenya. As a matter related to gender roles, this religious official rightly identifies that male clergy are effective in delivering religious pronouncements in making people aware of the theological dimensions of HIV and AIDS, whereas women living in religious communities in Eastern Africa are providing direct care and support for the human being, living with this medical condition. Together, both efforts can be effective in treating the whole person, body and soul.

The distinction between male and female efforts by Catholics responding to HIV and AIDS in Nairobi may also reflect certain gender roles governed by culture as well as by religion. "Many of the women will have the virus but they don't know they have it," stated another Catholic leader engaged in prevention efforts. "This is because of migratory labor, their husband moves down to Mombasa or up to Nairobi and when he is there he moves around, and so he can come back with the virus and the woman is not aware that he has the virus."[18] Migratory labor is but one of the major reasons for increased rates of infection—along with long-distance truck drivers and members of the military—who are away from their families for extended periods of time and who then engage in transactional sex.[19]

Regarding the place of the wife, the respondent continued, "[the wife] is not aware that she has the virus until she gets sick. And of course, if she bears a child and she doesn't know she has the virus because the antenatal care is just too far away. So she just simply goes through her pregnancy with the help maybe a mid-wife sometimes to talk to." There is an inherent imbalance between the wife and husband in this scenario, since the wife "gives birth, and nobody knows if the child has the virus or not because she doesn't know she has the virus."[20]

This tragic development calls into question the fidelity of married people and the theologically and culturally grounded norms associated with prescribed gender roles in Kenya. Stated interrogatively, why would the wife need to be tested if she believes that her husband—to whom she made wedding vows of fidelity—had remained faithful? Raising again the issue of incorporating realistic human behavior into the Church response to AIDS, voluntary counseling and testing (VCT) is an important element in disease prevention since it provides individuals with knowledge of their status before engaging in sexual intercourse. Fear remains for many in actually knowing their infection status due to the various ways the disease is transmitted and how they will be treated by their friends and family if the test results are positive.

Reflecting on the serious challenge of societal explanations regarding entrenched notions of gender and disease transmission, the topic of promiscuity is controversial. The bias, historically in favor of men, is evident in the words of the Catholic educator on being promiscuous. "I think, for a man, the society will be more forgiving. For a woman, they are not that forgiving. They are not very kind. So women and men are judged on very different standards. There is a double standard."[21] This double standard in judging how men and women act sexually is not only religiously conditioned, but it is also the product of Kenyan popular culture:

> I mean, it's like a man having an affair. Somebody will say, "Anyway, it's just typically a man. It's typical male behavior. What's the big deal?" Somebody will say, "My father had three, four, five wives. So why shouldn't I?" You know, it's very easy to dismiss it. It's like it's part of masculine behavior but not feminine behavior. So women are judged much more harshly than men would be judged. So there's that gender dimension to it.[22]

Given this disparity between how men and women are expected to behave sexually, gender roles of masculinity and femininity are tempered by prevailing notions of sexuality identified by this respondent as stemming from patriarchal society. "Oh, it's from the patriarchal society. Basically, it comes from that society that—a lot of rules are made by men, and somehow they tend to favor the men. And the roles that we assume, women are supposed to be put in a box. You are supposed to behave this way."[23]

As a form of behavior regulation similar to stigma, this imbalanced set of standards on how men and women should act not only affects how HIV is transmitted—in the case of infidelity on the part of the man, unbeknownst to his wife—it also affects how those living with the disease understand it and seek treatment. The subject noted on the difference of how men and women approach being HIV positive, it "doesn't stop women from seeking help. Inasmuch as they are judged harshly, women would seek more help than men would. They would go to counseling, they would join a support group. If you visit a lot of our support groups, they are full of women. The men are not there. So again, the way you deal with it also is very gendered."[24] Considering the bias regarding the sexuality of women, there are definite cultural views pertaining to gender roles in Kenya which are indeed patriarchal. But again, there are biases in the theological traditions themselves going back to the Bible.

"So there is a lot of gender—if you look at how those issues are dealt with, it goes right back to the Bible," this Catholic interlocutor remarked, speaking from the voice of religious tradition. "You remember, the woman caught in adultery. You know the Bible clearly says they were caught, but it's only one who was taken in front—so I don't know where the man disappeared to," referring to the Gospel of John 8:4–11 in which Jesus is challenged by the Pharisees on what to do with a woman who was "caught in very act of committing adultery."[25] The subject continued introspectively on the man caught in adultery, "[t]he Levites are not really interested in what, to deal with the man. They were more interested. . . . Like he didn't do wrong, but she did wrong. So, very gendered—it has very deep historical and biblical roots. It didn't start now. It started then."[26]

Probing the biblical roots of gender inequality, this respondent identifies the inherent imbalance of church patriarchy as something that women have had to live with for some time, even independent of the HIV and AIDS epidemic. The crisis itself can be understood as magnifying the social structures that have led to further infection in Kenya including the very gender roles that are promulgated within the religious communities. At their very core, gender roles involve what is expected from men and women—influenced by culture and religion—which can make HIV prevention and treatment that much more difficult. "It has to do with masculinity. You know, hospitals they normally say are women's spaces. You know, women are always taking children to hospital," continued the subject. "But for a man, [the hospital is] not a place—he really goes when he's very ill. And a man, even if you're sick you're not supposed to show it that easily. So men grow up kind of thinking a sign of sickness is a sign of weakness."[27]

Speaking from obvious experience, this Catholic leader sees that established ideas regarding acceptable masculine behavior overshadow even self-preservation, since men are not supposed to betray symptoms of illness. When this notion of masculinity is directed toward HIV and AIDS in Nairobi, the result is tragic with men infecting women because they themselves either don't know they are HIV positive or they don't want to be seen as sick. With either scenario, silence intensifies the disease. The subject continued, "[s]eeking out help is—I can do it on my own. But it ends up working against them. It's all these concepts of masculinity—you are the decision maker . . . otherwise it's down to consult a counselor to tell me how to lead my life. What can another man or a woman for that tell me how to behave or how to treat my wife?"[28]

With this rugged sense of individualism and independence, men who are advised to undergo VCT often feel threatened. This instinctive reaction can be attributed to the fear of actually knowing their infection status. Providing health care, prevention initiatives, education, and destigmatization efforts can prove difficult in the face of such adversity, particularly among the male population. In the words of this particular leader, patriarchal society and dominant roles of masculinity can "sometimes interfere" with church efforts in responding to the AIDS epidemic. "But women because I think they are ready to listen, they are always being told, so they can seek out advice. It's not a less—it doesn't make you less if you reach out for help," the subject concluded. "But I think for the men it might be they feel, it makes you feel less, you know, when you seek out help. You'd rather just deal with the issue yourself, even if it's killing you."[29]

This evident disparity of the sexes once again makes efforts in health care and prevention much more problematic since the men in this subject's assessment possess no desire to seek help. While this is a sweeping generalization, there may be some merit to the assumption that men feel as though they don't need to seek help, VCT, or treatment for fear that they might be losing some status in negotiating the power dynamic between the sexes. Stigma mitigation as it relates to gender roles and the perception of risk of contracting the virus, assumes a much deeper dimension since Catholic relief workers are forced to address overarching notions of entrenched gender biases as well as combatting prevailing convictions about HIV transmission. As the subject noted, men in Kenyan society might not seek out medical help, "even if it's killing you." If these men are unwilling to find help or take part in VCT to know their status, this increases the overall threat to others. In this way, biased gender roles serve to undermine AIDS prevention efforts by the Catholic Church, which is, again, itself based on a patriarchal framework and hierarchy.

One area of recourse can be found in an unlikely source, the Kenyan Constitution which was ratified in 2010. This document proposes life goals for all Kenyan citizens, among them freedom from past discrimination (§27.6); the establishment of the national Human Rights and Equality Commission which focuses on gender issues (§59.2.B); the elimination of gender discrimination in law, customs, land and property (§60.1.F); eliminating gender inequality in political parties (§91.1.F and §91.2.A), among many other provisions.[30] This Constitution establishes a basic standard toward which the country continues to strive, with the goals still attractive in their ends.

On the aims of the document and its lasting effect on the broader Kenyan society, one Catholic leader remarked, "I think personally is that one of the goals [of the Kenyan Constitution (2010)] is to eliminate gender-based violence and to bring equality, reduce the disparity between the genders. And the Constitution is safeguarding the rights of everybody. People are now more aware about their rights, and where to go if your rights are violated."[31] In this candid formulation about the impact of the newest iteration of the Kenyan Constitution, gender is indeed an important topic in the national discourse.

Even where Catholic leaders are reluctant to speak about the depth of importance in dealing with normative gender roles, the government has made significant advances in addressing the disparity between the sexes, reified by religion and culture. Said the interlocutor, bringing into the discussion elements of gender in relation to health care, "with the Constitution ensuring that you have access to such things as credit and money, and education—universal education—for all. You see, it is uplifting the standards of everyone. So it somehow has a spillover effect on so many other things, even health care."[32] In a surprising move, this discussant looked to the mechanisms within society that allow for the inequality of the sexes and how the Constitution of 2010 serves to address many of the areas of concern identified in this project—namely, HIV and AIDS prevention, education, and destigmatization.

That the government of Kenya should engage issues such as gender, inequality, education, and health care is worth consideration since, from a religious perspective, speaking about such topics can be sensitive. "So the Constitution, I think everybody knows—it's unlike before, you're out on your own. And if nothing comes to you, there is nothing you can do. Now, at least you have—you know that there is a government that cares and they are doing A, B, C, D to try and sort out most of welfare issues," the subject concluded. "So people are much better off now with the Constitution and their rights are being better safeguarded. Yeah. And the disparity between the men and the women, I think is—you know—it's really sorting that out."[33]

The political developments enshrined in this Constitution have given the population of Kenya a decided advantage in addressing and combatting much gender inequality from a legal perspective—though these provisions themselves may prove difficult to actually enforce. Nevertheless, Kenyan Catholics now have a secular, political channel for facing the lasting challenge of gender bias. Though it may take some time, Catholics in Nairobi are confronting the very real challenge of entrenched gender roles in their everyday lives partially in terms of religion and partially in terms of society and politics. The cumulative effect, as this relates to the AIDS crisis, is that people are self-consciously questioning the status quo and are moving ahead to transparently seek help and information about the virus in order to deconstruct perceptions of power and dominance as this relates to the concepts of gender in contemporary society—including the problematic issue of condom use in HIV and AIDS prevention.

Catholics Speaking about Condoms

Simply stated, condom use is a very difficult theological issue to negotiate. While much has been written in Catholic moral theology, even on the distinction between condom use as prophylaxis and contraception, the presence of condoms in the debate about HIV and AIDS has proven problematic from a practical standpoint.[34] The life-giving act of sexual intercourse must never be prevented, as Pope Paul VI notes, so the use of contraceptives is intrinsically evil and immoral since "excluded is any action which either before, at the moment of, or after sexual intercourse, is specifically intended to prevent procreation—whether as an end or as a means."[35]

Yet, as an integral way of preventing disease transmission, condom use while not 100 percent effective remains a proven way to combat HIV infection. Even PEPFAR's ABC's include the use of condoms as a method of disease prevention, though relegated to the third position behind abstinence and staying faithful to your committed partner. This framework and methodological tool does not, however, provide any recourse to those who, under the heading of Catholic moral theology, make mistakes—those that do not abstain, the couples who are not faithful, and those who do not use condoms with multiple partners. While each of these acts are themselves mortal sins, a practically realistic approach might be necessary to combat the spread of HIV and AIDS in Kenya, one that acknowledges that humans are prone to making mistakes and commiting sins. Prevention efforts based in a theology of forgiveness may bear fruit where moralistic judgment has engendered silence.

Reflecting on the impact on gender roles and even the implicit power dynamic between man and woman, which can be found also in industrialized Western countries, one Catholic respondent offered the insightful observation that, "I can't ask my partner, if I'm a woman, I can't ask the guy to wear a condom. And I can't say show me a letter saying that you've been tested and that you are negative. You follow? So there's that risk. And that's very nearly where poverty compounds the transmission."[36] In this realistic assessment, the subject identifies several of the cultural factors leading to virus transmission in Nairobi, chief among them the imbalance of power in intimate relationships, basic concepts of gender roles and their negotiation in daily life, and even poverty have led to HIV infection in the city.

In this mundane portrait of Catholic life in Nairobi, PEPFAR's ABC's of AIDS prevention don't always apply. "Also, I mean from the point of view of getting access to medical care, if I'm in these communities when—I talk for the woman—because they're the often head of the household," the discussant continued. "I wake up in the morning and my first concern is whether there will be food for the family? Getting the child to school—yes I want to try to get the child to school, but if I have no money to buy whatever, I have to pay whatever—that's a problem."[37] Hinting at the tragic decision that many women throughout the world face on a daily basis, each of these prevention measures—abstaining, staying faithful, and using condoms—does not address the root causes leading to AIDS infection and the unbalanced power dynamic between men and women.[38]

In addition, income disparity continues to be a very real concern for half the world population living under the international poverty line, many of whom live in Eastern Africa. In fatalistic terms, the subject concluded that, "Clothes are not such an issue in this country because they are available for very small prices—and we don't need that number of clothes, like in the developed world. But going for medical care, if I have an opportunistic infection then I can pass away because I don't get the medical care that would have kept me alive."[39] This subject speaks to the basic necessities of life—clothing, education, and medical care—as a constant challenge for those living in Nairobi with HIV. With an average per capita income of $1,800, providing medical care for people living with HIV and AIDS in the form of antiretroviral therapy remains prohibitively expensive for the most vulnerable poor.[40] Those left untreated are susceptible to opportunistic infections such as cholera, typhoid, and pneumonia.

This lived scenario for millions of Kenyans is further compounded by the fact that these individuals need to provide basic necessities such as clothing and shelter for themselves and often for their entire families as well. As this subject rightly acknowledged, "poverty compounds the transmission."[41] What is necessary are social structures in place that allow those living with the disease at the lowest socioeconomic level to achieve their full human potential, toward which many within the Catholic leadership are already working. And yet condom use remains one of those neuralgic issues that certain religious leaders cannot see past, from both within Islam and Catholicism.

"You see because we then sort of share this common opposition. So [the Muslims] have responded to issues of use of condoms. They have responded to issues of education curriculum, that the government has designed. Basically opposing it, just as the Catholics have," attested one Catholic priest living in Nairobi. "I'm not familiar with how much happens under the Muslim banner at the grassroots level. I do know that at the level of advocacy, there have been some significant positions that have been adopted, led by Muslim leaders—usually the imams."[42] This priest clearly addresses the shared opposition of both Muslim and Catholic leaders to the government's curriculum on AIDS education and prevention, which advocates condom use among people who otherwise would choose to have unprotected sex with multiple partners.

That these religious leaders stand in opposition to condom use is an interesting interreligious development as there is a broad range of views on the matter, even within the Catholic religious tradition. Though, from a strictly theological standpoint, the use of condoms or any method that would prevent the sexual act from producing children, is prohibited and considered objectively a mortal sin. As the *Catechism of the Catholic Church* states, citing *Familiaris Consortio*, no. 32:

> Thus the innate language that expresses the total reciprocal self-giving of husband and wife is overlaid, through contraception, by an objectively contradictory language, namely, that of not giving oneself totally to the other. This leads not only to a positive refusal to be open to life but also to a falsification of the inner truth of conjugal love, which is called upon to give itself in personal totality. . . . The difference, both anthropological and moral, between contraception and recourse to the rhythm of the cycle . . . involves in the final analysis two irreconcilable concepts of the human person and of human sexuality.[43]

This excerpt considers the legitimate aims of conjugal love, addressing the similarities between the human person as both anthropological and moral being. The Catechism later states, "legitimate intentions on the part of the spouses do not justify recourse to morally unacceptable means (for example, direct sterilization or contraception)."[44]

Yet, even with this explicit injunction on the use of contraceptives, there are those Catholic leaders who use theological principles to justify the use of condoms in prevention efforts especially between serodiscordant couples. "Well, the use of condoms obviously is a question with theological implications, right? So there are two well-proven theological principles which speak to that. And that is the principle of the double effect and the principle of the unjust aggressor. So both of them apply to the use of a condom," offered one Catholic official, referring to these two prominent principles in moral theology.

While an extended analysis of these two principles is beyond the scope of this section, a brief overview may prove helpful. In the church teaching on the unjust aggressor, it is licit from a theological standpoint to repel violence with violence in defending life, property of importance, and chastity—"even to the extent of killing an unjust assailant. This is admitted to be true with the reservation included in the phrase, 'servato moderamine inculpatæ tutelæ.' That is, only that degree of violence may be employed which is necessary adequately to protect one from the attack."[45]

Since the principle seeks to maintain self-preservation through self-defense, the use of a condom by someone who knows they are HIV positive may indeed prove licit. The subject explained, "[t]he unjust aggressor, that you have to protect yourself if you're positive. Because if you have sex with another person who is positive then you will, their mutation will be transferred to you and yours to them. So there's an unjust aggressor element."[46] In this formulation, using a condom during sexual intercourse is not necessarily a form of contraceptive, but rather serves as a form of prophylaxis—preserving the human physical organism from the risk of initial or discordant infection. "And if—like in the case of our young person—he would have had to use a condom all the time, except when they were endeavoring to conceive a child so to protect his partner who is negative," further stated the Catholic official on discordant couples, where one is infected or is infected with a different strain of the virus.[47]

The second principle, that of double effect, needs some clarification. A central tenet of Catholic moral theology is the exhortation to pursue good and avoid that which is bad or evil.[48] The ethical principle of double effect allows Catholics to evaluate the moral dimensions of theologically challenging issues, which themselves cause unintended consequences—both positive and negative. Double effect governs actions that are morally good but may carry negative consequences, in this case the use of condoms to prevent virus transmission, thereby saving life. "Just as morphine can be used to kill a patient and/or to alleviate a patient's pain, similarly a condom in a marriage in which one partner is infected and the wife is not post-menopausal can be used to prevent the transmission of HIV and/or to avoid a pregnancy," write Fr. James. F. Keenan and Dr. Jon D. Fuller, SJ. "Though the possibility of a contraceptive effect can be foreseen, it cannot be intended. And just as a patient in pain is not denied pain relief in light of a foreseen but unintended effect, neither should a married couple be denied protected conjugal love even though the protection could be contraceptive."[49]

Though the principle of double effect has several more parameters—such as guidelines to judge whether an action is morally acceptable—the central premise assumes that some moral acts result in negative consequences and that these guiding conditions can determine whether an action is licit or illicit. The subject continued, "double effect is, we're using the condom not for contraception which is the double effect but for protection."[50] In the case of condom use for discordant couples, employing the principle of double effect does make some sense, since the moral position seeks to prevent further transmission of the disease—and not necessarily to prevent a child from being born.

While the issue then becomes one of motivation in both cases, the end result is the preservation of human life. As a practical matter, many Catholic leaders seek to use their theology and its moral principles to assure that the needs of those living with the virus are being addressed, responding pastorally in the face of opposition from other members of the clergy. "So that is—

the position of the hierarchical church, of the institutional church, is that the condom is—is forbidden in the Catholic Church, let me say," confided the respondent.[51] This self-conscious assertion exposes the various views regarding HIV and AIDS prevention, as well as the opposition that many working in the field face as they attempt to use their confessional religion to make sense of the epidemic treating those living with the virus, both theologically and practically.

In a candid example of theology and praxis coming at a crossroads, the subject remembered, "[t]he late Archbishop here in this country spoke about [condom use] in the context of discordant couples. . . . He spoke about that and he was very much reprehended by the other bishops of the country. There is a bishop down in South Africa who speaks very openly about that. They are the ones I know because I'm in Africa."[52] Even in the face of censure by other members of the Catholic community, there are those leaders and care providers who strive to illuminate the question of condom usage within their own theological traditions. Breaking down stereotypes and working to change the popular opinion about the virus throughout the city and the country, these officials offer a form of triage for persons infected as well as for those who are at risk of becoming infected.

This seems to be the heart of the issue—that no practical prevention efforts by the Catholic Church can proceed effectively without first addressing the root causes of the debate over condoms. With the wide range of views on the matter, the general population of Kenyan Catholics must equally be polarized with both secular and religious information on the subject of condoms and disease prevention. Yet there are those courageous leaders who challenge the status quo in the hopes of preventing future infection by arguing for the adoption of condom use as an effective means of preventing HIV transmission. This is not, however, to accept condom use wholesale with no restrictions. In the words of the Catholic official serving in the area of grassroots advocacy and prevention, "[n]ow, the whole issue of condom, that has to be—[Catholic Church leaders] need to become enlightened about that, of the fact that the use of it in discordant couples is absolutely essential."[53]

Though leaders struggle in advocating for the use of condoms among married, faithful, discordant couples, the wide breadth of official and personal opinions about condoms can be a difficult issue to resolve. In the lived Catholic response to HIV and AIDS in Nairobi, one educator offered that, there are some things "that you kind of really tread really carefully. You know things like homosexuality. Because there is no common ground. And you know condom use."[54] This section concludes with the quotation to offer an uneasy and incomplete picture of HIV and AIDS prevention as this relates to condoms. Theologically, there is absolutely common ground on the topic of condom use—that they are prohibited because they prevent life. Practically, however, there still remains a gray area in which Catholic leaders continue trying to break down barriers so they can provide care to those living with and those who are negatively affected by the AIDS epidemic in Nairobi.

Other Catholic Views on Sexuality and Condom Use

It might be evident at this point that the present research project promotes a progressive view toward the three areas presented above that does not coalesce fully with other orthodox views from within Catholicism. Therefore, it would be disingenuous at this point to neglect to acknowledge that there are drastically different views in moral theology pertaining to the controversies of sexual intercourse, gender roles, and condom use stemming from the AIDS epidemic in Nairobi. That is, there are very real, explicit disagreements about each of the three areas identified in this chapter on sexuality within the Catholic Church—not only in Kenya but throughout the world and involving all levels of church authority, from the grassroots to the Vatican.

As noted elsewhere, the principal strategy for the Church in preventing the spread of AIDS has been an emphasis on abstinence and fidelity which goes down to the very heart of Christian theology and the ends of human sexuality. "It should be noted here that the concern of the Churches is not simply with the health message of avoiding HIV, but also with the theological message being true to the meaning and purpose of human sexuality," writes Fr. Michael J. Kelly, SJ. "Even if there were no risk of HIV transmission, the Churches would not countenance premarital sex or any form of marital infidelity, since these involve departure from central principles of behavior based on the Christian understanding that being sexual is constitutive of what it means to be human."[55] Fr. Kelly's assertion—that even if there were no threat of HIV in the world, the Catholic Church would still continue to promote abstinence and fidelity—bears further consideration as humans often fall short of what is expected of them by church doctrine and teaching.

For example, while traveling through Africa in 2009, Pope Benedict XVI sought to clarify the Catholic Church position on HIV prevention in a twofold manner. First, responding to AIDS throughout the world calls for a "humanisation of sexuality and a true friendship, especially for those who are suffering."[56] While church prevention efforts based in personal responsibility and human sexuality have had a profound impact in understanding and curbing transmission of the disease from a theological perspective, there are still those who contend that fidelity and abstinence both are ineffective and unrealistic for preventing the spread of HIV. This is perhaps why a single focus on abstinence and fidelity faces such hostility from those that deal with the practical impact of the virus in their own religious communities.[57]

Second, Pope Benedict stated that the distribution of condoms would not resolve the issue of AIDS but, in an interesting move, he asserted that their presence might actually make matters worse. Although secular media outlets focused on the negative impact of this statement, they generally overlooked the formal doctrinal teachings of the Church on condom use. The official church teaching on condom use as expressly forbidden is unambiguous, as seen in the preceding discussion of *Humane Vitae*, based in "the first principles of a human and Christian doctrine of marriage," that "the direct interruption of the generative process already begun and, above all, all direct abortion, even for therapeutic reasons, are to be absolutely excluded as lawful means of regulating the number of children."[58] The document further states:

> Neither is it valid to argue, as a justification for sexual intercourse which is deliberately contraceptive, that a lesser evil is to be preferred to a greater one, or that such intercourse would merge with procreative acts of past and future to form a single entity, and so be qualified by exactly the same moral goodness as these. Though it is true that sometimes it is lawful to tolerate a lesser moral evil in order to avoid a greater evil or in order to promote a greater good, it is never lawful, even for the gravest reasons, to do evil that good may come of it—in other words, to intend directly something which of its very nature contradicts the moral order, and which must therefore be judged unworthy of man, even though the intention is to protect or promote the welfare of an individual, of a family or of society in general. Consequently, it is a serious error to think that a whole married life of otherwise normal relations can justify sexual intercourse which is deliberately contraceptive and so intrinsically wrong.[59]

Humane Vitae thus addresses many of the moral arguments made at the beginning of this chapter on the permissibility of condom use. Quite simply, sexual intercourse outside of marriage is intrinsically wrong, as is the use of condoms for "deliberatively contraceptive" purposes.

And yet even with the document's authoritative voice, while explicitly forbidden, the discourse surrounding condom use in preventing HIV and AIDS transmission remains a controversial matter between the various mechanisms, institutions, and bodies that make up the Catholic Church:

> Condoms make for a contentious issue for many of the Churches. A polarizing debate about their use has bedeviled prevention work almost since the onset of the pandemic. For the greater part, FBO's have been portrayed as opposing condoms and secular public health organizations as being in their favour, although the picture is not quite so sharp for PEPFAR, the US President's Emergency Fund for AIDS Relief. Several considerations appear to motivate Church concerns about the condom: their dual role for contraceptive and therapeutic use; the impression sometimes conveyed that unrestricted condom use is the best way to prevent new HIV infections; the concern that having recourse to a condom could undermine an authentically human sense of sexual-

ity; the way using a condom may be interpreted as a means of protecting oneself against HIV while making no change in the sexual practices that put one at risk of infection; the possibility that the indiscriminate distribution of condoms would lead to increased sexual activity outside of or prior to marriage; and the false sense of security that condoms can engender even though they are not one hundred percent effective in preventing HIV transmission.[60]

Even as secular public health experts formally acknowledged that the use of condoms could be an effective strategy for preventing AIDS in the early days of the worldwide epidemic, the Catholic Church maintained its official policy prohibiting their use. "There is no Church statement, however, comparable in authority with that of *Humanae Vitae*, banning the use of condoms for this therapeutic purpose of preventing the transmission of a highly infectious and frequently fatal disease," Kelly writes. "Instead, official statements repeatedly take the positive approach of proclaiming abstinence and the proper understanding of Christian sexuality as the safest and most principled methods for avoiding HIV transmission."[61]

This is where the discussion of abstinence, being faithful, and condom use comes full circle and their relationship to each other are further clarified by church teaching. Whereas the unmarried are called to remain abstinent and the married are called to stay faithful to each other, the use of condoms in the discussion of AIDS prevention from the highest levels of church authority is explicitly forbidden. This is not to say that there are not discrepancies and disagreements about how the official church strategy is enacted and policed in the various dioceses and parishes of the world, but also on a much more interpersonal level, the discussion highlights the tense relationship between doctrine and practice that results in various beliefs, practices, and teachings—particularly in relation to AIDS.

"If we are sufficiently uncomfortable with perplexity, we simply hold on to the insights that have served us well, and we avert our eyes from alternatives that might otherwise force us to change course. Yet moral and religious insights have a way of growing or fading," writes Margaret A. Farley. "They become deeper and more nuanced, or they are vulnerable to rigid, even fanatic distortions of their original truth. Hence, when we probe apparent contradictions and unsatisfying ambiguities, sometimes we come to better insights, clearer perceptions of the content of our moral obligations."[62] Even with the various secular public health initiatives at work in contemporary Kenya, condom use in HIV and AIDS prevention does not provide absolute protection from the virus—a point often overlooked by media outlets and popular views regarding the epidemic.

Indeed, as Farley notes, there are those Catholic leaders who do distort their original truths—truths indoctrinated and promulgated for centuries. "Justice necessitates truth," Michael Kelly affirms. "But the truth about condom limitations and the success of the church prevention approach is not always fully communicated. This is an injustice."[63] This assertion once again highlights the intersection of official church teaching and how this teaching is contextualized in a particular social setting.

Thus, whereas controversies related to abstinence, being faithful, and even condom use remain in a tense balance between teaching and daily life, given the depth and breadth of opinion between Catholic leaders and lay practitioners, there should be little wonder that certain elements of church teaching remain inviolable. While the Catholic Church is often criticized over its position prohibiting condom use in preventing HIV and AIDS transmission—instead stressing abstinence and remaining faithful as the only absolutely effective means of disease prevention—as a religious institution and the moral compass of a significant percentage of the worldwide population, these differences of opinion might actually help to clarify the underlying official church teaching and official positions, which can then inform and motivate all those who are responding to those living with HIV and AIDS, from the leadership to the laity.

Conclusion to Catholics and Sexuality

"At the grassroots level, the women they just want to get people taken care of," affirmed the Jesuit leader living in Kenya's capital. "They are not worried about the ethical issues, should you be use a condom or not, for example,; what about discordant couples? Can you do 'ABC'? They have found, they have made their peace with those controversies."[64] As a concluding statement, this priest provides a remarkable estimation of how church magisterial teachings and the everyday life of Kenya's Catholic meet at a crossroads. Whereas there are official church policies and doctrines related to life as it is daily lived for the Catholic population of Nairobi, there is a degree of flexibility in how this teaching is enforced and promulgated. Indeed, those living with the virus are being treated by Catholic health-care providers without intrusive moral judgment because there is a need to do so.

As the Jesuit notes, certain segments of the Catholic population—particularly those working at the grassroots level—see past the conceptual hurdles in order to provide appropriate care and treatment for those living with HIV infection. The urgency of the matter is something that Catholic leaders throughout Kenya must deal with realistically and practically. Making peace with these controversies allows for an actual engagement with the society within which the Catholic Church lives and operates, while distancing themselves from the troublesome issues that pose theological roadblocks such as condom use. As advocates of social justice and grassroots activism, those Catholic leaders and officials providing care and sustenance to local communities are truly performing God's works—through mercy, hospitality, and justice among other religious virtues—helping to save and transform lives negatively affected by this debilitating medical condition.

On this apparent disconnect between official church teaching and grassroots advocacy, the priest elaborates, "Where I saw the level, the official level, we tend to get stuck on these ethical questions around prevention, and sexuality, and all of that. I see that as a big difference."[65] This last point helps to clarify the discussion of all three points addressed in the first section of this chapter and brings to light issues pertaining to sexuality, gender roles, and condoms in a fairly succinct passage. Instead of engaging in a theological debate over whether the use of condoms to prevent HIV is moral or immoral, women religious working at the grassroots level "just want people taken care of."

It is the women, then, who are deconstructing gender roles, talking about sexuality, and putting to rest the moral questions surrounding condoms in order to actually provide care for those living with the virus. Women engaged in advocacy and activism in the above account are more concerned with providing effective health care, education, and stigma mitigation rather than debating over the Catholic Church's official position on controversies such as which methods can or cannot be used to prevent HIV infection.

A final word on the impact of sexuality on the Church response to AIDS from the perspective of a Catholic nun who lives and works in Nairobi. When questioned about her hopes for the future of HIV and AIDS prevention in Kenya, she responded quite self-consciously, "I would hope that the pastoral aspect of Jesus' message would now have the prominence, and that sexuality would come into a much more balanced context in the Church's teaching. That's what my hope would be."[66] The issue of sexuality, long influencing Catholic efforts in education and destigmatization including the ABC's of AIDS prevention for this religious care provider still needs to be addressed—both theologically and practically.

"But, now you see, the doctrinal aspect of the Church also has been emphasized considerably versus the actual pastoral ministry. So I'd hope that the balance there would also—because the doctrine was the last word," the Catholic nun continued. Reflecting on the tension between church doctrine and actual pastoral care for those infected with the virus, she concluded, "Whereas if you look at the gospels, you see Jesus—Jesus didn't relate with people according to formal doctrinal position. He related from compassion. It didn't mean that he didn't challenge, but compassion was an overriding dimension in his whole approach to people."[67]

That Jesus's approach to people was steeped in compassion and mercy instead of magisterial doctrine is a profound point, one which this nun clearly uses to move past the controversies over condom use and patriarchy so that she can embody the compassion she so clearly sees in Jesus's dealings with his fellow humans. On this topic, the nun cleverly offered a rejoinder, which brings the interview full-circle on the topic of HIV in Nairobi, saying, "I hope that that balance [between sexuality, doctrine, and pastoral care] will happen. That will affect the whole issue of HIV as well."[68]

Issues of sexuality—among them sexual intercourse, gender roles, and condom use—remain contentious for the Catholic Church and for church leaders working in the strategic areas of HIV prevention, education, and destigmatization. From the official to the grassroots, there are many different voices and opinions on how to best respond to the AIDS epidemic in Kenya's capital city, particularly for those who are negatively affected by the virus. And, though advances have been made in these three strategic areas since the early days of the outbreak in Kenya, there is still much work to be done both officially and pastorally. These tensions are not exclusive to Catholicism in Nairobi, but rather manifest themselves in the Muslim community as well.

Muslims Speaking about Sexual Intercourse

"So another thing I want to add, because according to Qur'ān teachings, Allah says "*Wala taqrabu zina.*" Do not approach adultery or fornication," asserted one imam in Nairobi. "That is enough. So that means, do not approach—you have to take care."[69] The imam is speaking of the Qur'ānic injunction against adultery and fornication in Surah *Al-Isra*, which states, "And approach not fornication; Surely it is an indecency, and evil as a way."[70] This command, based in the authority of God's revelation to mankind in the Qur'ān, came up in several interviews as a matter of shared belief and conviction. In a move that resonates with the PEPFAR's ABC's of AIDS prevention, another imam working on Islamic curriculum development in Nairobi advanced, "the most important thing in Islam is just to make sure that you abstain before getting married, you avoid those types of immorality or whatever. And if you are married, then be faithful to your partner."[71]

While this interlocutor addresses the PEPFAR's A and B—to abstain and be faithful—the issue of condoms was referenced significantly less as a means of prevention. Nevertheless, abstinence and spousal fidelity are themes common to Islam and Catholicism. The imam then takes the discussion in an interesting direction, addressing a point of contention between religion and culture—Islam's sanction for allowing for more than one wife. "And this, we are asked why we have been given a chance to marry more than one [wife]? Why?" he asked rhetorically. "Because if you tell me only to marry one wife, maybe I will need another one. But the rules are not allowing me to do so, then I have to ban fornication. So unlike other religions Islam is somehow open to matters of the woman. So the most important thing in Islam is to abstain."[72]

The imam highlights that, even with the provision in the Kenyan Constitution (2010) providing for Islamic *khadi* courts who have jurisdiction over family and inheritance laws, Islamic law takes a secondary position to civil law and that any sexual relations outside of recognized marriage is unlawful.[73] Therefore, those who have not yet married must abstain from engaging in any sexual activity as proscribed by the Qur'ān. As a matter of common conviction, another sheikh echoed the same sentiments when he affirmed, "If you're not married. If you are married then stay faithful to your wife. You keep yourself from things that will lead you [to commit *zina* (Arabic, unlawful sexual intercourse)]. For example, in Islam a girl or a youth is not allowed to wear maybe a short skirt or tight clothes—maybe men would get some temptation. And then it will lead you to *zina*. So that's prevention."[74]

Making the conceptual leap from theology to its practical application, the Muslim leader sees curbing sexual temptation—in the form of reinforcing standards of modest dress—as an important element in preventing disease transmission. This jump from scripture to everyday life is one which helps clarifying just how sexual intercourse and disease transmission can be addressed in the daily lives of the Muslim population of Nairobi. In a practical example, another imam reflects on the lived impact of *zina* on the population, in realistic human terms. "Remember, we usually talk about the evil of *zina*. And we say that the effect of *zina* is not HIV only," he explained. "Children, unwanted children. Maybe now, especially in Kenya, we have—I think you have seen a lot of street children. The majority of them are from *zina*. Because the woman had a baby that was an unwanted child. So his father, or her father disappeared. Now, it's the mother only."[75]

In an account similar to the Catholic perspective highlighting the emphasis on HIV and sexuality—particularly from the imbalanced gender perspective of Kenyan culture—sexuality may be difficult to speak about from a religious perspective particularly because of its inherent power dynamic. When questioned on how HIV is understood from within the specifically Islamic religious tradition, the imam offered the following reflection, again highlighting the relationship between religion and society as informed by culture. "We understand HIV/AIDS the way you understand it, as a disease. That you can get it in so many ways," he stated. "You can get it yourself from unprotected sex with a person who is infected. But what we as Muslims believe that not each and every person infected by HIV is a wrong one." Considering further the imbalance between the sexes, on the topic of sexual intercourse, the imam continued, "You might be faithful to your wife, but she is not faithful. So she goes out, she does her own thing and she brings HIV in the house."[76]

This movement from theology to practical life—embodied in the belief that people can transmit the disease through having sex outside of marriage—does draw a narrow focus on sexual relations and disease transmission, betraying a criticism levied also by women religious of the Catholic theological tradition. Additionally, it allows for an acknowledgment of realistic human behavior informed by a theology that allows for forgiveness. "So Islam—the way other people understand HIV is the way we understand [it]. Because the HIV that affects them is no different than the HIV that affects us," the speaker observed. On the randomness of infection probability and moving away from a specific focus on AIDS and sexual intercourse, he concluded, "Also you can get it through an accident. Maybe you get injured and the other person there, you share blood. So you can get it there."[77]

This account moves past sexuality into a discussion of how the virus can be transmitted in alternative ways—among them in many East African nations mere chance and culture. Yet the popularly perceived manners of transmission, those of disordered sexuality or promiscuity, do remain. "I remember, before 10 years in Malindi—you know Malindi? A girl got—she was infected by HIV through ear-piercing. So wanted to get married, she was a virgin," said the sheikh. "But when she tested, she got that HIV infection. So they wondered. Nobody maybe had sex with her, and she got that disease. So they knew that when she went there for ear pierce, so she got that infection."[78] This recollection demystifies the narrative that HIV can only be transmitted through sexual intercourse. That a girl can contract the virus through having her ears pierced is telling, since historically the infection has been contracted through any number of ways—from untested blood transfusions, to circumcision ceremonies, even through a haircut.[79]

And yet this virgin who contracted the disease through no fault of her own is still forced to address issues of sexual transmission among other contemporary factors such as culture. "There are certain cultures, for example, initiation in the beach and also in the fish industry. The lady when she wants to work in that area then she needs to be initiated. Therefore she has to sleep with the man," explained one Muslim sheikh on the tension between culture and Islam. "So there are certain cultures. And the trend you will see, for example, in Nyanza the infection will be higher because of certain cultures. And also Meru because of certain cultures. There are other financial issues."[80] Intimating at the prospect of sexual expectations and transactional sex that, as a tragic yet stark reality, does occur even within religious communities. "For example," the subject continued, "in Nyanza because the fisherman have cash flow, a lot of cash flow on a daily basis. So they have a lot of money to spend. And they believe, also, which is also a part of culture is that you have to spend today's money so that you can get another one tomorrow."[81]

Regarding the impact of culture on sexual relations and HIV—particularly in communities where transactional sexual intercourse is dependent on scarce resources that are only available for short periods of time, such as in the fishing villages in Nyanza—the Muslim speaker offers the insight that these fishermen in Western Kenya opt to spend the money they make every day because, "Otherwise, if you save you will not get any more. Or maybe you will feel lazy, because I have money I don't have to work. So if you don't have money, it's a motivation to work so that you get money."[82]

Culture, then, has a large influence on how HIV and AIDS is spread, not solely from a religious perspective, this observation also exposes how sexual intercourse is perceived throughout Kenya. In a very practical sense, disease transmission is complicated due to numerous factors, not least of all due to the nexus of culture and religion. Islamic leaders are therefore faced with an essential challenge—how to address HIV and AIDS as a lived reality as religious officials within their own religious communities. On this scenario, one imam offered the following reflection, "we use our pulpit, our mosque, our member—we sensitize youth. So another case, maybe someone has been affected from the HIV. What we do, we encourage them to use medicine to take ARV, and they do need patience."[83]

As a religious leader and a member of the Islamic community of Nairobi, the imam plays an integral role in how the broader community comes to terms with the disease as well as how they understand how it is transmitted, how it is treated, and the risk of contracting the disease. Also addressed is the view that HIV infection may be a test from God. For example, the Qur'ān states, when the believer is confronted with fear, hunger, and the "diminution of goods and lives and fruits," God will "give good tidings unto the patient who, when they are visited by an affliction, say, 'Surely we belong to God and to Him we return'; upon those rest blessings and mercy from their Lord, and those—they are the truly guided."[84]

The imam continued, "I know some couples maybe the wife is faithful, but the husband maybe has got that disease from elsewhere. So maybe the husband passed away, now we try to assist the widows and the orphans and we tell them to be patient and to take medicine."[85] Highlighting the lasting influence of gender roles, which will be considered in the subsequent section, this Muslim leader offers a realistic account of what happens when a member of the Islamic community of Nairobi admits they have the disease. Knowing their status and coming to terms with it, the religious community, as well as the Muslim leadership, can then offer support where it is needed in the form of advocacy, VCT, monetary support, medical care, and otherwise. He concluded, "[t]he most important thing in Islam, if you are not married then abstain. If you are married, be faithful."[86]

Reiterating the adopted script that closely resembles the ABC's of AIDS prevention, this imam raises both the theological and actual implications of HIV and AIDS within the Muslim community—that the epidemic is a test from God, and those affected and infected must remain patient and faithful. However, given the religiously and culturally entrenched gender roles, the discussion takes on an interesting trajectory to which we now turn.

Muslims Speaking about Gender Roles

"Well there is a lady, one time we were several years ago, we were trying to sensitize ladies to—Muslims women—to come out and speak out [about their condition]. We did a program called 'Behind the Veil' with another Muslim sister," recollected one prominent imam who preaches in a central mosque in Nairobi. "And there's a lady who read an *ayat* from the Qur'an that says, 'Which of the favors of your God would you deny?' And according to her, she said 'HIV and AIDS came to me and found me on the prayer mat.' "[87] Such an intimate portrait serves to show just how disease transmission is understood and accepted by the Muslim community. Far from being a punishment from God—as it is often understood by some—this woman self-consciously accepted that she had contracted the disease and, as such, must live with it as a chronic medical condition.

"That the husband might have contracted HIV and AIDS outside there, and therefore infected her," the imam continued. "So it's not that she went out or she went to hospital or anything or contracted it through means that are well-known. But she believed that it was through the husband."[88] Once again, the issue of gender roles plays an unmistakable place in the discourse on HIV and AIDS prevention, education, and prevention. That the husband in this specific case contracted the disease in what would seem to be adulterous circumstances demonstrates the imbalance of gender at the forefront of the conversation.

Yet, the woman in this instance resigns herself to the fact that HIV infection found her on the prayer mat. Instead of staying silent, she sought comfort in her faith and from within the Muslim community. The imam self-critically interjected, "[s]o that statement, that *ayat* that says 'Which of your Lord's favors do you deny?' made me, left me thinking that 'Well, this—whatever God blesses you with. Whatever situation you find yourself in, it could be a big favor from God.' And therefore, one—you cannot deny it."[89]

This is a very powerful example, one which illuminates the imbalance of gender in the discussion of HIV and AIDS in Kenya and actually seeks to radically redefine how those living with infection are accepted by the Muslim community. As a test, people living with the disease can use their religion to understand the medical condition as a blessing—God chose them because of the strength of their faith and that not as a punishment for disordered behavior. However, for many Muslims, having contracted the disease has led to an increased disparity between the genders, made worse by several factors—such as transactional sex, modernity, and physiology.

Poverty can lead people to engage in transactional sex, one sheikh acknowledged that one of the main reasons HIV transmission continues even after Muslim efforts in health care and prevention, is poverty. Said one subject, "if you have no food, someone comes—maybe there is no food in the house—someone comes, gives her five hundred shillings. Of course, because she is in need of the money, she'll have to do what the guys wants. Poverty's the first thing."[90] In this grim estimation, the woman is forced to accept money for sex acts, reinforcing dominant ideas regarding gender referenced earlier with its connection to culture. Poverty therefore makes gender roles further imbalanced thereby increasing HIV risk.

Referring to another area of concern regarding disease transmission and gender roles, the sheikh identifies collective morality and the lack thereof. "Then secondly, immorality—lack of values from our parents and leaders. Now, before our fathers used to tell us that they were being guided from a young age until they were getting married."[91] This clear guidance from families and leaders within the Muslim community in Nairobi had been historically defined in terms of values and morals. "But nowadays," the sheikh concluded, "when a child reaches 15, we tend to believe now he is free to go to do everything he wants. So immorality, poverty, lack of clear guidance from our leaders and families."[92]

Of course in the above account, the Islamic leader offers his analysis from the perspective of the male adolescent, leaving out the female who may experience these influences differently. Yet, his observations on the continued spread of HIV from within the Islamic population of Nairobi shows some insight from the perspective of someone who has seen a shift in how Muslims approach the disease. The issue of morality and how it can be infected by notions of gender is a fascinating topic, one which many respondents address in relation to modernity. After all, negotiating Islamic identity in a cosmopolitan city such as Nairobi can be difficult, especially for youth who are confronted by advances in such areas as technology.

"Another thing you can add maybe to morality, interaction between males and females," added another Islamic official at one of Nairobi's largest mosques. "Also, another thing I think, you can say films. Our youth watch on the TV dirty movies, films. Now they can download pornography on their phones."[93] While the interaction between males and females in the form of pornography is not a new sociohistorical development, the way this imam conceptually shifts to the ability of youth to download videos and images onto their smart phones betrays a distrust of modernity, especially as this relates to sexuality and gender roles.

Nevertheless, in maintaining and affirming the central importance of sexuality in committed and officially recognized marriages, the imam shares concerns about sexual temptation in Nairobi. In negotiating their Islamic identity in the face of modernity, adolescents in this capital city are also dealing with the inherent gender roles established both religiously and culturally.

One concluding point on how physiology affects gender roles in Nairobi may be in order. Due to the advances in education, prevention, and destigmatization discussed elsewhere in this project, many Muslims are relatively well-educated on the biomedical dimensions of HIV and AIDS transmission from a practical, physical standpoint. "Women are more affected by HIV than men," rightly stated one Muslim educator. "I think religiously, I don't think Islam has anything to say about it. Because it's about physiologically. Because it's about the physical creation of the person."[94]

The sheikh is correct that women are disproportionately affected by the epidemic, not only in Kenya but throughout the world.[95] This is partially true because of culture—such as dominant gender roles, which do not allow women to ask their intimate partners to wear condoms and even infidelity in marriages—but much of the problem of disease transmission stems from the physical nature of the female reproductive organ which is much more prone to tearing than the male organ.[96] Given that women bear the onus of the gendered worldwide infection rate, there are medical procedures that men can undergo to reduce their risk of infection as well as their risk of infecting their sexual partners.

Take, for example, voluntary male circumcision which has proven an effective method for preventing HIV infection.[97] On this topic, the sheikh continued, "we know that in Kenya we have had this campaign where now men from a certain part of the country are going under circumcision, because they never used to do it. It was not part of their culture."[98] Reflecting on the nexus of culture, religion, gender, and physiology, the subject proposes that the efficacy of voluntary male circumcision in preventing AIDS infection is beginning to prompt certain cultures to change their customs, saying: "Now they are doing it because it statistics have revealed that they are more prone to HIV and AIDS because of the foreskin. So they cut it."[99] The sheikh then offered a medically correct view of human anatomy, "The physiology of a woman is such a way that it is easy for her to cut, to have HIV and AIDS. Because she receives. Because we know that not all of those who have engaged in sex outside of marriage have contracted HIV. And maybe they have had sexual relationships with people with HIV and AIDS."[100]

Acknowledging that there are many different ways to contract the virus, this subject makes the stark point that not everyone who engages in high-risk behavior acquires the virus. He concludes, "it just depends on the way that that was done. I think that its just that we cannot as a religious community, you cannot condemn one group or say that one group is more at fault in terms of HIV and AIDS. It's physiological."[101]

As an issue at the crossroads of culture, society, and religion, the influence of established gender roles in Nairobi plays a prominent part in the Muslim discourse surrounding HIV and AIDS prevention, health care, education, and destigmatization. The basic power imbalance between the sexes has made efforts in these areas all the more challenging and problematic, as Islamic leaders strive to identify and clarify the internal dimensions of the gender dynamic so that they as religious officials can provide better information, care, and treatment options to those living with the virus in Nairobi. Where these sheikhs and imams negotiate gender roles in relation to modernity, advances have been made in familiarizing themselves with the biomedical and bioethical aspects of the disease so they can provide scientifically correct and medically proven advice to those infected throughout Kenya's capital city. While much work remains, these Muslim leaders are adapting their strategies for dealing with the epidemic in Kenya, which even involves condom use.

Muslims Speaking about Condoms

As a matter of disease prevention, condom use is a contentious issue. From this research, several Muslim interlocutors posed practical aspects to the problem of condoms—prominently, the role the government plays in its overarching prevention efforts, the concern over how to adapt to modernity at the university level, and finally the religious constraints based in scripture that Muslim leaders face when speaking to their congregations about HIV prevention and transmission.

When questioned how living in the metropolitan center of Kenya has impacted his religious self-understanding, one imam remarked, "you fall prey to a lot of other bad things. So for us we say, 'You know, the government should be strong enough in terms of acting on situations that encourage or lead to certain situations that might lead to HIV and AIDS infection.' "[102] Considering the role the government plays in shaping public opinion and behavior, the promotion of condom use in disease prevention becomes one of popular perception that then raises the issue of condom advertising and marketing in Nairobi. "And even the condom issue—and this is from an Islamic perspective—and I believe I have worked with the Catholics and even from that perspective, that even the way they advertise the condom, they make it look to young people like it's a very nice thing," said the imam, emphasizing the influence that advertising has on how the population of Nairobi views the use of condoms from a secular perspective.

However, a religious official charged with leading and instructing the Muslim population of the city mentioned that such marketing sends mixed signals. "As religious people, we try to work on abstinence more than prevention in terms of using a condom," the imam reflected. "So we say that even the way the advertise the condom looks like a very nice thing, and therefore some people would be tempted to want to use it."[103] This temptation directs itself to our basic human instincts. In this imam's estimation, the advertising and availability of condoms leads to the commodification of sex—a view anathema to Catholic Church and Islamic teachings.

Also, a major fault this Muslim leader has with these government objectives in prevention is, while they may make condoms seem appealing, they don't actually teach people how to use them. "And they don't know, they don't have the knowledge on how to use [the condom]—good knowledge," said the subject. "And people get infected because they did not use it properly. So these are some of the things."[104] The above reflection, while it does carry some ethical and moral bearing in Islamic teaching and scripture also raises a practical pastoral command—if people are going to use condoms for whatever reason, they should be taught how to effectively use them so that they can prevent much disease transmission.

A fascinating development, then, is the imam's directed conversation toward community activism related to the government's position on condom use. "In terms of our response as a community, well it is lacking. It has been lacking," he noted. "Apart from what I mentioned, a few responses here and there, it's totally lacking."[105] And yet, the question persists as to how is the Muslim population—and specifically within that segment of the population of Nairobi, the Islamic leaders, sheikhs, and imams—are meant to challenge the strategic aims of the national and municipal government in disease prevention through marketing condoms.

To conclude his interview, the imam offered the introspective thought on community activism, saying, "maybe it's time for the community to start saying, 'No. HIV and AIDS is also an issue, and we have to talk about it very, very loudly so that people know.' "[106] Though there are those Islamic organizations that take part in grassroots advocacy and activism in Nairobi—such as SUPKEM and the KCI—it can be difficult to maneuver the complex relationship between religion and society. Another area not often referenced by the Islamic leadership as a means of disease transmission—that of IDU—remains an area of concern for many Muslims. One imam identified the government's efforts at intravenous drug use have, in fact, had the very opposite effect. "You know brother, it goes vice versa," he said. "From some point nowadays, the government announces every time about how it has been effective about drug abuse. But they see an increase—every time."[107] The imam is speaking about the trend that, for at least the past decade, the Kenyan government has seen a steady increase in the use of intravenous drug use, such as heroin, in its capital city during the last decade.[108]

Though secular governmental efforts have sought to educate IDU's on the potential for contracting the disease through injection with dirty needles, the statistic continues to rise as the imam notes. As a matter of external consequence from the perspective of the Kenyan government, the imam offered his insight, citing that people, "want to test, so they test that drug. If you announce every time, 'Don't use. Don't use.' Youth want to try."[109] Thus, the activity of the government in HIV prevention efforts in the areas of condom distribution and IDU reduction have actually and unintentionally served to make matters worse. On the topic of human nature, the imam offers the concluding remark on the connection between secular advertising and drug use, "Yeah, [the government statistic on drug users] has gone up every time. You know, our problem is that the youth want to try everything. So if you keep on advertising this thing, they want to do it. How does it taste?"[110]

The element of temptation, evident in the past two interviews, remains difficult to fully address from the Islamic perspective since, as this latter subject asserts, advertising and marketing directly involve the question of "how does it taste?" In the opinion of these religious leaders, the government is actually making the social situation for Muslims in Nairobi worse by inadvertently providing temptation, though the efforts are meant to prevent disease transmission. When asked to assess the present social situation in the city, one prominent sheikh offered, "[i]n my personal opinion? Ok, in my personal opinion, I think the government has tried fighting HIV. But it was using the wrong avenues if you keep on advertising these condoms."[111]

Considering the tense relationship between the government and the Muslim population, these Islamic leaders see that the efforts by the Kenyan government have targeted the wrong root causes of the epidemic. Similar to his colleagues, the subject criticizes the secular prevention objectives as misguided, addressing the symptoms of the epidemic instead of addressing the root causes of the disease. He further stated on the influence of centers of higher learning such as the university setting, "If you go to these public universities, there is a special place for condoms. The message is that you are free to do sex, as long as you use thing. Ok, condoms—I think the government has tried. It has tried, but not to the level that the government should."[112]

Identifying the tension between the secular government, the secular public universities, and Islam in the discussion of HIV prevention, this subject offered a critical picture of the government's aims in responding to AIDS with its overemphasis on condoms as the most effective means of preventing disease transmission, even distributing them freely throughout public universities in Nairobi. With such an intense focus on condoms—and their clear association with sexual intercourse—Muslim leaders show concern over the commodification of sex at the university level where young, impressionable minds are met with culturally, ethnically, and religiously conflicting views on the status quo—both from an orthodox and liberal perspective.

"I think, the main reason to go to university is to gain knowledge. And for you to gain knowledge, you have to be someone who is responsible for yourself," asserted another imam on the major reasons why young people attend universities in Nairobi. This responsibility is not only directed to the individual Muslim going to college, but it also has a lasting effect on the Islamic community. He continued, "Because after a few years you are going to be a leader. So if you are a leader who always thinks of carrying condoms in your pockets, you are being brought up in an environment that tells you that you are free to do whatever you want."[113] The responsibility this imam references is contradicted by the education received at the university where condoms are accepted and distributed as an effective method of preventing HIV transmission.

The authority of those leaders—both secular and religious—who advocate for condom use is called into question by these Islamic leaders, who see their motives as irresponsible. "But in Islam, we don't encourage such things," the imam observed. "In Islam, we just abstain until you get married. If you get married, then be faithful."[114] In a move that echoes several other Islamic leaders interviewed for this project and the ABC's of AIDS prevention, this subject speaks of abstinence and staying faithful as the most effective means of combatting HIV transmission throughout Kenya. Yet, where this imam stresses the A of "abstinence" and the B of "be faithful," he takes exception to distributing condoms to prevent disease transmission. As the imam concluded, "the issue of condoms, spreading them to hospitals, putting them here and there—I think it encourages *zina* and fornication, and that more than anything else. It's like saying it's good for you to do it so long as you use this. Just use it and you are free to do this [sexual intercourse]."[115]

Whether the presence of condoms in hospitals and universities in Nairobi, illuminated by government marketing and advertising, actually increases sexual activity among youth is a hotly debated topic. One concluding voice in the discussion of condom use and *zina* helps to bring us full circle, this imam involved in VCT programs and education from the Islamic position, offered the view of scripture as illuminating the actual impact of condoms use in disease transmission, stating, "[t]he Qur'ān, Allah told us—He did not tell us not to fornicate. He told us, 'Do not come close to, do not approach.' And when sheikhs—the scholars—try to explain that, they say, 'Do not come to anything that will lead you [to *zina*].' "[116]

Thus, citing the Qur'ānic mandate of Surah *Al-Isra* 17:32, to "not approach unlawful sexual intercourse," the Muslims of Nairobi are instructed not to come close to anything that would lead them to sexual acts inappropriate or illicit in the established Islamic order—such as fornication or adultery as well as the use of condoms. By preserving Islamic identity in the face of cultural and social change, these leaders are teaching their congregations about the risks of becoming infected, rooted in Islamic scripture though heavily informed by a realistic understanding of human nature. Said the imam, "by the time you reach there [approaching *zina*]—you can say, 'Well I can be in a room with a lady and nothing will happen.' But we are always told that if you are locked in a room for twenty-four hours with a very ugly lady, at some point she will become very pretty. You will start seeing the pretty in her."[117]

While clearly referencing some of the other issues that lead to an imbalance of gender roles as this relates to the AIDS epidemic in Kenya, the above example offered by this imam gives a human face to the scripture on why humans are drawn toward committing *zina*. By extension, this example can also be applied to the presence of condoms in the debate over prevention of future infection. "So do not come close. So those items like condoms, like whatever—let's not even go closer to that because they will lead us into more disastrous situations," affirmed the imam. While the practical implication of such a view is open to much debate particularly in terms of prevention, the theological significance returns to abstinence and fidelity as the only completely effective means of preventing infection, not only in Kenya among Muslims but throughout the world. The imam concluded, "As human beings, God knows that we cannot really control ourselves in certain situations. So that is an explanation of that. Do not come close to *zina*. . . . Anything that might lead to *zina*, to committing adultery."[118]

This understanding of scripture as providing the most effective prevention of HIV transmission is noteworthy since, at the very heart of the issue, condoms are not a cure for the disease but rather are a stopgap maneuver from infecting other people. "It's not a cure," said one sheikh. "And you're not even 80% that it will prevent you from HIV."[119] As this subject notes, the fact remains that using condoms will not provide a remedy for the AIDS epidemic in Nairobi but will rather only keep the disease at bay at the present moment. Returning to the ABC's of AIDS prevention, nearly all the Islamic subjects interviewed cited abstinence and remaining faithful to your intimate partner as the most effective and legitimately sanctioned by religious scripture such as the Qur'ān. "So, I think that if we stay on the rule of being faithful to your wife or whatever, and abstain if you are not married—things will change," the sheikh conjectured. "Instead of just encouraging, use condoms. You make condoms as if to be the cure."[120]

CONCLUSION

At the intersection of secular society and religion, Catholics and Muslims in Nairobi have been presented with the challenge of negotiating their self-identification in light of complex and often conflicting factors. Religious leaders in both communities of faith are thus charged with responding in an official capacity to the pressing concerns facing their respective communities, both theologically and practically. Particularly since these religious groups do not operate in isolation but are in may ways adaptive to their society, priests and nuns, imams and sheikhs are responsible for addressing the needs of their religious faithful—including those living with HIV and AIDS infection.

One troublesome issue that remains at the forefront of secular and religious debate on the topic of AIDS in Nairobi is that of sexuality—both in general and specifically in three areas. As this section presented, the matter of sexuality remains an area of contention—not only between the government and religions, but also intra-religiously. Many religious officials do not know how to actually speak about physical human sexuality in realistic terms. What is necessary is a theology based in compassion and forgiveness, one that acknowledges that humans will make mistakes—that they will not abstain, that they will not always remain faithful to their committed partners. Or, in the prescient words of one imam who preaches in Nairobi, "if somebody was infected from *zina*—so he has to repent to Allah to seek forgiveness and pardon. And we believe that Allah will forgive him."[121]

On the topic of sexuality, these religious communities need open places to speak about sexuality, both in the mosque and the Church, as well as within civil society in an atmosphere that does not carry moral judgment on how the disease has been contracted. In this section, the research has identified three specific areas of present concern in the discourse surrounding the HIV and AIDS epidemic in Nairobi from both the Catholic and Sunni Muslim vantage point: sexual activity, gender roles, and the issue of condoms.

First, sexual activity remains an area of tension due to the extreme focus on sexual intercourse as the sole method of disease transmission. While it is true that sexual intercourse is one way of contracting the virus, the common mechanical reaction from both Muslim and Catholic leaders serves to overemphasize the place of sexuality in the discussion of HIV and AIDS prevention. Such a focus does not address other factors of disease transmission. The cumulative effect of this belief is that sex is the single identifiable source of infection.

Second, the culturally and religiously perceived and promulgated ideas surrounding gender roles of masculinity and femininity make speaking about HIV and AIDS difficult topics to breach. This is in part due to the fact that Kenyan men are not expected to admit that they have been infected, nor to seek treatment when they begin to show symptoms. From the perspective of the female population, women have little power to dictate their own role in their sexual lives. This can lead to further infection as they cannot force their partners to use a condom or to question their partner's fidelity. Some women religious—specifically within Catholicism—are working to deconstruct and break down these established gender roles so that they can provide practical and religious support to those living with infection, irrespective of religious self-identification, gender, or ethnicity.

Third, the issue of condom use in the debate over HIV prevention remains theologically clear yet practically murky. On the one hand, from both within Catholicism and Sunni Islam in Kenya today, the use of condoms as a contraceptive is prohibited in all cases as religious leaders opt instead to emphasize abstinence and fidelity as the most effective means of disease prevention. Yet, as the Catholic nun explains in the present chapter, making the conceptual switch from condom use as contraceptive to its use as a prophylaxis—preventing infection and preserving life—using the Catholic moral principle of double effect, some religious leaders struggle to make sense of how to treat persons living with AIDS in terms of theology while also seeking to prevent future infection.

What remains is a portrait of Kenya's capital as a modern and urban city, yet one which still clings to its religious roots and institutions. There is still much work to be done—especially in illuminating the role of sexuality in the shared religious response to HIV and AIDS throughout Kenya. Muslim and Catholic leaders over the past thirty years have adapted their roles as both pastoral and religious caregivers so that they can serve those people living with infection in Nairobi in order to respond both theologically and practically to those in need.

NOTES

1. The opening quotation from this chapter comes from the Holy Bible, John 8:7.
2. Lisa Sowle Cahill, *Bioethics and the Common Good* (Milwaukee, WI: Marquette University Press, 2004), 76.
3. Ibid.
4. Given that the issue of sexuality is disproportionately identified by the wider Kenyan public as a major factor in the continued spread of HIV and AIDS, I here tried to steer clear of an overemphasis on this particular topic, as has been discussed elsewhere in the project. However, given the prominence of sexuality in the interview material, it would be irresponsible to not bring it up in this chapter on lingering questions and largely unaddressed concerns.
5. Cahill, *Bioethics and the Common Good*, 67.
6. Personal Interview—Nairobi, Kenya, 6.13.14.
7. Messer, *Breaking the Conspiracy of Silence*, 104–11.
8. Personal Interview—Nairobi, Kenya, 6.20.14.
9. Ibid.
10. Ibid.
11. Ibid.
12. Ibid.
13. Personal Interview—Nairobi, Kenya, 6.13.14.
14. Ibid.
15. Ed. Judith Worell, *Encyclopedia of Women and Gender: Sex Similarities and Differences and the Impact of Society on Gender*, Vol. 2 (Waltham, MA: Academic Press Publishing Company, 2001), 645.
16. Personal Interview—Nairobi, Kenya, 6.18.14.
17. Ibid.
18. Personal Interview—Nairobi, Kenya, 6.20.14.
19. Marian Burghardt, "Subjects of Counselling: Religion, HIV/AIDS and the Management of Everyday Life in South Africa," in *AIDS and Religious Practice in Africa*, 341.
20. Personal Interview—Nairobi, Kenya, 6.20.14.
21. Personal Interview—Nairobi, Kenya, 6.13.14.
22. Ibid.
23. Ibid.
24. Ibid.

25. Bible, John 8:4.
26. Personal Interview—Nairobi, Kenya, 6.13.14.
27. Ibid.
28. Ibid.
29. Ibid.
30. *Constitution of Kenya*, articles referenced above.
31. Personal Interview—Nairobi, Kenya, 7.3.15.
32. Ibid.
33. Ibid.
34. See Kenyan Episcopal Conference (KEC), "The Church Speaks and Teaches," in *This We Teach and Do: Catholic Church and AIDS in Kenya*, Vol. 1—*Policy*, 27; eds. James F. Keenan, Jon Fuller, SJ, Lisa Cahill, and Kevin Kelly, *Catholic Ethicists on HIV/AIDS Prevention*; Messer, *Breaking the Conspiracy of Silence*; Kelly, *HIV and AIDS: A Social Justice Perspective*, 237; ed. Becker and Geissler, *AIDS and Religious Practice in Africa*; Cahill, *Bioethics and the Common Good.*
35. Encyclical Letter on the Regulation of Birth, *Humanae Vitae* (Vatican: the Holy See, Rome, 25 July 1968), §14. The issue of contraception is also taken up by Pope John Paul II in Apostolic Exhortation on the Role of the Christian Family in the Modern World, *Familiaris Consortio* (Vatican: the Holy See, Rome, November 22, 1981), §30–32.
36. Personal Interview—Nairobi, Kenya, 6.20.14.
37. Ibid.
38. Jo Sadgrove, " 'Keeping Up Appearances': Sex and Religion Amongst University Students in Uganda" in *AIDS and Religious Practice in Africa*, 230–36.
39. Personal Interview—Nairobi, Kenya, 6.20.14.
40. CIA, "Africa—Kenya," 8.
41. Personal Interview—Nairobi, Kenya, 6.20.14.
42. Personal Interview—Nairobi, Kenya, 6.18.14.
43. Catholic Church, *Catechism of the Catholic Church*, § 2370.
44. Ibid., § 2399.
45. Eds. Charles G. Herbermann, Edward A. Pace, Condé B. Pallen, Thomas J. Shahan, and John J. Wynne, SJ, *The Catholic Encyclopedia: An International Work of Reference on the Constitution, Doctrine, Discipline, and History of the Catholic Church*, Vol. 1 (New York: The Encyclopedia Press, Inc., 1913), 210.
46. Personal Interview—Nairobi, Kenya, 6.20.14.
47. Ibid.
48. Catholic Church, *Catechism of the Catholic Church*. On this topic, §1732 reads, "As long as freedom has not bound itself definitively to its ultimate good which is God, there is the possibility of *choosing between good and evil*, and thus of growing in perfection or of failing and sinning. This freedom characterizes properly human acts. It is the basis of praise or blame, merit or reproach." Also, see § 1954, which reads, "Man participates in the wisdom and goodness of the Creator who gives him mastery over his acts and the ability to govern himself with a view to the true and the good. The natural law expresses the original moral sense which enables man to discern by reason the good and the evil, the truth and the lie."
49. James F. Keenan, SJ and Jon D. Fuller, SJ, "Condoms, Catholics and HIV/AIDS Prevention," *The Furrow* 52 (2001): 462–63.
50. Personal Interview—Nairobi, Kenya, 6.20.14.
51. Ibid.
52. Ibid.
53. Ibid.
54. Personal Interview—Nairobi, Kenya, 6.18.14.
55. Kelly, *HIV and AIDS*, 231.
56. Ibid.
57. Cahill, *Bioethics and the Common Good*, 67–75.
58. *Humanae Vitae*, §14.

59. Ibid. For an extended exploration of several controversies concerning human sexuality from a feminist perspective, see Margaret A. Farley, *Just Love: A Framework for Christian Sexual Ethics* (London, UK: Continuum International Publishing Group, 2006), 215–32.
60. Kelly, *HIV and AIDS*, 233.
61. Ibid., 234.
62. Farley, *Compassionate Respect*, 3–4.
63. Kelly, *HIV and AIDS*, 236.
64. Personal Interview—Nairobi, Kenya, 6.13.14.
65. Ibid.
66. Personal Interview—Nairobi, Kenya, 6.20.14.
67. Ibid.
68. Ibid.
69. Personal Interview—Nairobi, Kenya, 6.19.14.b.
70. Qur'ān 17:32.
71. Personal Interview—Nairobi, Kenya, 6.19.14.a.
72. Ibid.
73. *Constitution of Kenya*, §24.4; §161.9.b; §170.1–5.
74. Personal Interview—Nairobi, Kenya, 6.19.14.c.
75. Personal Interview—Nairobi, Kenya, 6.19.14.b.
76. Ibid.
77. Ibid.
78. Personal Interview—Nairobi, Kenya, 6.19.14.c.
79. Rijk van Dijk, "Gloves in the Time of AIDS: Pentecostalism, Hair, and Social Distancing in Botswana" in *AIDS and Religious Practice in Africa*, 290–94.
80. Personal Interview—Nairobi, Kenya, 6.12.14.
81. Ibid.
82. Ibid.
83. Personal Interview—Nairobi, Kenya, 6.19.14.a.
84. Qur'ān 2:155–57.
85. Personal Interview—Nairobi, Kenya, 6.19.14.a.
86. Ibid.
87. Personal Interview—Nairobi, Kenya, 6.17.14.
88. Ibid.
89. Ibid.
90. Personal Interview—Nairobi, Kenya, 6.19.14.c.
91. Ibid.
92. Ibid.
93. Personal Interview—Nairobi, Kenya, 6.19.14.b.
94. Personal Interview—Nairobi, Kenya, 6.19.14.c.
95. UNAIDS, 16.
96. Ibid.
97. Ibid., 18–20.
98. Personal Interview—Nairobi, Kenya, 6.19.14.c.
99. Ibid.
100. Ibid.
101. Ibid.
102. Personal Interview—Nairobi, Kenya, 6.17.14.
103. Ibid.
104. Ibid.
105. Ibid.
106. Ibid.
107. Personal Interview—Nairobi, Kenya, 6.19.14.b.
108. Steffanie A. Strathdee, Timothy B. Hallett, Natalia Bobrova, Tim Rhodes, Robert Booth, Reychad Abdool, Catherine A. Hankins, "HIV and Risk Environment for Injecting Drug Users: The Past, Present, and Future," *The Lancet* 376 (24 July 2010), 275.
109. Personal Interview—Nairobi, Kenya, 6.19.14.b.

110. Ibid.
111. Personal Interview—Nairobi, Kenya, 6.19.14.c.
112. Ibid.
113. Personal Interview—Nairobi, Kenya, 6.19.14.b.
114. Ibid.
115. Ibid.
116. Personal Interview—Nairobi, Kenya, 6.19.14.a.
117. Ibid.
118. Ibid.
119. Personal Interview—Nairobi, Kenya, 6.19.14.c.
120. Ibid.
121. Personal Interview—Nairobi, Kenya, 6.19.14.a.

Conclusion

"Therefore, the Lord waits to be gracious to you; therefore He will rise up to show mercy to you. For the Lord is a God of justice; blessed are those who wait for Him."

INTRODUCTION TO THE CONCLUSION

One basic assumption motivating this research project is that religions interact with the societies they inhabit in certain observable and describable patterns that can then be compared.[1] While this manuscript focused on how Muslim and Catholic leaders are addressing the HIV and AIDS epidemic in Nairobi, Kenya, it is my hope that the present study has highlighted the productive ways those most influential actors—namely, Muslim and Catholic leaders in Kenya who respond to the crisis and the *kairos* of AIDS in daily life—have introspectively reflected on not only their own efforts in responding to HIV and AIDS infection in their own communities, but also how their respective religious representatives and religious institutions have responded historically and recently, both for the worse and for the better.

"Serious moral and religious obligations are always more complex than we think they will be. Ethical guidelines and theological concepts are stretched at every turn, even in our ordinary lives," begins Catholic ethicist Margaret A. Farley in her 2002 Madeleva Lecture in Spirituality entitled, *Compassionate Respect: A Feminist Approach to Medical Ethics and Other Questions*. "What seems sufficient at one time in our personal and social histories is all too soon challenged by new situations or evolving and sometimes conflicting experiences. One conviction, insight, or internalized moral norm is countered by another, so that perplexity threatens to derail our efforts at moral discernment."[2]

Following from Farley's assertion above, the AIDS epidemic throughout Kenya represents a perplexing experience to those negatively affected by the virus, and this is perhaps why the HIV and AIDS religious discourse is such an interesting lens with which to view the practical response to AIDS and those living with the virus in Nairobi. As an interlocutor who is an outsider, I am not constrained by political affiliations, religious self-identification, socioeconomic status, or personal history in the city. Rather, I can observe and report as a theologian who struggles with the reality of HIV and AIDS in Kenya, albeit in markedly different ways. Instead of objectively quantifying each religion's efforts in the areas of prevention, education, and destigmatization, this work offers a descriptive account of the struggles and achievements of these Catholic and Muslim leaders working in Nairobi in their own voices—voices that remain largely unheard outside of their immediate social milieu and context. These religious leaders are attempting to articulate their roles while theologically coming to terms with the HIV and AIDS epidemic in their own religious communities while being faced daily with the practical necessity of attending to the needs of their faithful congregations who are negatively affected by the disease.

As this epidemic concerns the comparative religious responses to the AIDS epidemic in Kenya, this study has focused on the following religious yet practical issues: on education, misinformation about the virus and its transmission continues to be disseminated even though factually correct information is available; on prevention, the disease continues to spread even though Catholic and Muslim officials and health-care workers serve the common good in their tireless efforts at curbing infection; and on stigma, discrimination continues even though both religious traditions teach that each of us has an intrinsic dignity common to all. The work by these men and women of faith aims to affirm the inherent, inherent value of the human person—irrespective of religious self-identification or HIV status—through their common acts of mercy, hospitality, and justice.

THE AIDS EPIDEMIC AND THE INTERRELIGIOUS RESPONSE

Perhaps this commonality is why religious officials, such as this local Catholic educator, are compelled to conjecture, "even for me, as a Catholic working here, I think ecumenism is a wonderful thing in the modern society. Because you work with other people, you understand each other more when you interact with them." The subject continued on the reality of religious differences, "If you are brought up in one faith, only mix with other people of one faith, go to school with only one faith then that suspicion will always be there, them and we—or us. And what are these differences? You realize that there are very artificial boundaries that separate us."[3]

The critical self-reflexivity displayed by this subject addresses the very real threat of HIV and AIDS infection that has forced leaders in Nairobi to reassess and reidentify their own notions of religious practice and identity as fellow Kenyans who feel the immediacy of responding to this epidemic, which carries both social and physical implications. That this particular interlocutor acknowledges many of the boundaries religious persons construct are artificial is worth considering further, since officials from both Islam and Catholicism have come together to respond to the actual needs of people living with infection, specifically in the identified fields of prevention, education, and destigmatization in the form of an organic interreligious dialogue.

Responding to what he perceives as differences in approaching HIV and AIDS care from within both religious traditions, one sheikh offered the view that, "I think that if there are any differences, then they are very little differences. Because among the advantages we have now is that there are lots of interfaith forums where we exchange ideas, exchange information." These exchanges have not only affected education, as evidenced above with the exchange of information, but also in terms of sensitization toward people from different faiths. Continued the sheikh, "Sometimes I am also invited in a church to give our Islamic response to something. And we borrow beliefs from each other. So in general, I don't think there's much difference."[4]

On the lasting impact of these interfaith forums where Muslims and Christians come together to exchange ideas and beliefs, the Muslim leader concludes, "at these forums, religious leaders—they exchange views and they give information. These are very important forums so that they grasp the right information, then they give it down to the community." And perhaps most importantly, "when you reach just one pastor or one sheikh or one imam, then you are reaching to so many people—five hundred, five thousand people at our congregation."[5]

The significance of sensitizing religious officials is evident in this account since these leaders hold much sway over public opinion, both religiously and socially. This is why the current manuscript seeks to document the voice of religious leaders on the topic of HIV and AIDS in Nairobi, specifically because of the considerable influence that these individuals have on popular views. "So the religious leaders tend to carry more credibility or attract credibility from people than would a political leader. And some of this is born out by actions that are undertaken by religious leaders. And when they advocate for issues of peace, reconciliation, justice, political transparency, etcetera—they are able to sort of fill in as a step in the bridge," added one Catholic priest on the positive impact of religious leaders.[6]

THE NEGATIVE LASTING IMPACT OF HIV AND AIDS IN KENYA

However, not every religious leader is inclined to act selflessly, working toward the common goods of mercy, hospitality, and justice. "I should say though this is not to gloss over the fact that there also have been instances—very disturbing instances—when religious leaders have been the ones fomenting some of these crises," the subject continued. "This, case in point, is the situation in Kenya today. And the influence of religious, I would say, fringe personalities who then incite people to violence."[7]

To paint too peaceful and settled a picture of contemporary Kenyan society would be naïve at best and irresponsible at worst. There have been many numerous cases of political, ethnic, and religious tensions at times boiling over into violence. From the 2008 postelection violence, to the September 2013 Westgate Shopping Mall bombing in downtown Nairobi, to the massacre at Mpeketoni while I was conducting my research between June 15 and 17, 2014, which left over sixty people dead in an apparent ethnic dispute, to the attacks against Christians at Garissa University College in April 2015—it is clear that many major practical issues must be confronted by both the government and religious communities of Kenya in order to address issues of national security.

And yet, even with these concerns over religious dysfunction, issues of HIV and AIDS remain at the forefront of national consciousness. "It is so necessary for the religious leaders to come together to address the common problem that affects each and every one in the community," asserted one Muslim official. "HIV does not discriminate based off anything. So it would be wise for us to come together as a community to fight the common problem for the community at large."[8] The HIV and AIDS epidemic throughout Kenya continues to be an area of great concern, not only within Catholicism and Islam, but also interreligiously.

CONCLUDING OVERVIEW

The overall aims of this project were manifold. Chapter 1 presented interview data collected during fieldwork to give voice to those Catholic clergy working at the crossroads of theology and religious practice in the areas of HIV and AIDS prevention, education, and destigmatization. It also made the conceptual distinction in each of these efforts of historically moving from crisis to *kairos*, God's appointed time for decisive action. This structure was largely adopted and adapted in chapter 2 for the Muslim perspective in the three areas noted above.

Chapter 3 extrapolated certain important theological traditions common to both Catholic and Islam with corresponding areas of practical activity: for prevention, mercy; for education, hospitality; and for destigmatization, justice. The concluding fourth chapter provided an overview of one of the major issues remaining in the interreligious discussion of HIV and AIDS in Nairobi—that of sexuality. Beginning with a discussion of sexuality, in general, from both a Catholic and Muslim perspective, the chapter then considered the impact of gender roles and condom use as areas of lasting concern over HIV transmission in Nairobi.

FINAL REFLECTIONS

One final reflection—a major impetus for this entire project stemmed from the belief that religions and persons religious occupy a unique position at the crossroads between faith and practice. Religions such as Sunni Islam and African Catholicism, their institutions, and leaders involve elements of both the human and the divine. Or, as one often quoted *Hadith* referenced in chapter 3 states from the perspective of God, "I was a hidden Treasure and I loved to be known: hence I created creation/human beings (*al-khalq*), so that I might be known."[9] All the universe—and by extension all of humanity—is contingent on God's divine love even though religious leaders and lay practitioners live out their faith in relation to other humans.

Humans, therefore, need God as well as other humans. From this, there is an intersection between the divine and the human dimensions of life since religion necessitates a human context. "Now you see, the doctrinal aspect of the Church also has been emphasized considerably versus the actual pastoral ministry," remarked one Catholic member of clergy. "Whereas if you look at the gospels, you see Jesus—Jesus didn't relate with people according to a formal doctrinal position. He related from compassion. It didn't mean that he didn't challenge [people], but compassion was an overriding dimension in his whole approach to people."[10] The leader concluded, "I hope that that balance between compassion and doctrine will happen. This will affect the whole issue of HIV as well."[11]

That Jesus himself was both man and Son of God presents a helpful model for bridging the gap between God and humanity. Similarly, in Islam, the Qur'ān and the Prophet Muhammad as the Messenger of God were able to cross over from the divine to the human world. This is why I posit that the HIV and AIDS epidemic in Nairobi is just such a compelling subject for theological analysis since it engages elements of both the body and the soul in relation to the whole person, raising such questions about pain, suffering, salvation, and ultimately death.

Catholic and Muslim leaders in present day Nairobi are called to work together in addressing and alleviating the pain of those living with infection, both theologically and practically. After all, the religious response, informed by the theological traditions of mercy, hospitality, and justice must be a form of social engagement—not just a theory, but an actual engagement—within the communities within which they are practiced. Specifically in the areas of prevention, education, and destigmatization, religious officials in both faith communities are increasingly being asked to serve as stewards of both the body and the soul all the while focusing on the place of mercy, hospitality, and justice in their efforts and strategic aims.

In conclusion, while the crisis of HIV and AIDS is the perfect time for God's decisive action—returning to the theological distinction of *kairos*—it also underscores the calling for a new strategy of Catholic and Muslim pastoral and medical care for those living with the human immunodeficiency virus and the acquired immunodeficiency syndrome by addressing the social context of the epidemic in Nairobi and responding appropriately to those in need.

By way of conclusion, I would like to address two elements of this project, one a central aim and the other a central concern. First, the central aim of this overall research is to bring to the forefront of theological discussion contemporary views on HIV and AIDS in Nairobi from the perspective of religious leadership in both Catholic and Sunni Muslim communities in Kenya's capital city. This was accomplished by interviewing nuns and priests, sheikhs and imams with the belief that these visible representatives of institutional authority hold significant influence over public opinion not only internally within their own religious congregations but also more broadly throughout the population of this East African country.

From this, programs aiming to target and educate the religious leadership are supremely important—as my interlocutors noted elsewhere in chapters 1 and 2—since radically redefining public opinion on infection and virus transmission have a profound impact on how Muslims and Catholics in Nairobi view the epidemic and those living with infection. Focusing on the representatives of religious authority, therefore, is an integral step in transforming the hearts and minds of both Muslim and Catholic communities in Nairobi.

Second, I concede a central concern. As a comparative theologian who chose to employ social scientific research tools for data collection, I made a conscious decision with significant effort to remain an unbiased observer and reporter of the views of HIV and AIDS from the religious leadership from within both Islam and Catholicism that I witnessed firsthand and recorded in Kenya's capital during the summer of 2014. This is, by all rights, a specific sociohistorical instance and the intra- and interreligious discourse will undoubtedly continue to adapt, evolve, and change to meet the demands of the present epidemic in order to affirm the inherent dignity of those living with the virus.

However, I now admit that for all of my efforts at remaining impartial, as a theologian concerned with the common good of society and with social justice in general, I have not produced an unbiased document or account of popular views of the AIDS epidemic in Nairobi. In the tradition of Margaret Farley, Michael Kelly, SJ, James F. Keenan, SJ, A. E. Orobator, SJ, and Lisa Sowle Cahill, there is no impartiality when it comes to AIDS. We as theologians and academics must take a stand in support of those living with the virus and those such as the families of those infected who are negatively affected by the epidemic in Kenya.

Thus, as a theologian with his own religious self-understanding, this project is weighted in favor of the positive elements of moral theology—those of justice, mercy, and hospitality. Indeed, as a researcher bringing my own story to the research, I self-selectively presented the views of those from the religious leadership that most closely resembled my own theology, one that favors a privileged place for those living with any form of illness not only in Kenya but more generally throughout the world.

After all, the first converts to both Islam and Christianity were among the marginalized—the sick, the elderly, the outcast, the downtrodden. And yet, these very same individuals were able to successfully and radically transform their own societies for the better in order to make them more equitable, fair, and just. As a clear example of the necessary move from crisis to *kairos*, so too are we now called not only as theologians, specialists, and academics but above all as members of humanity, in general, to be the impetus for a radical transformation of our own societies, moving ever closer to the community of believers that pride themselves on the traditions of mercy, justice, and hospitality.

It won't be easy and there are many institutional and artificial hurdles that stand in our way. But, if we are willing to creatively and dynamically redefine our own personal theologies in favor of one that provides a privileged place for those least well-off, in Kenya through the AIDS epidemic we can help to bring about a society within which all persons, including those living with HIV, can flourish and attain their own fullness of humanity.

NOTES

1. The opening quotation from this chapter comes from the Holy Bible Isaiah 30:18.
2. Farley, *Compassionate Respect*, 3.
3. Personal Interview—Nairobi, Kenya, 6.13.14.
4. Personal Interview—Nairobi, Kenya, 6.12.14.
5. Ibid.
6. Personal Interview—Nairobi, Kenya, 6.18.14.
7. Ibid.
8. Personal Interview—Nairobi, Kenya, 6.17.14.
9. Morris, *Openings*, 68.
10. Personal Interview—Nairobi, Kenya, 6.20.14.
11. Ibid.

Appendix A

Genesis 18:1–15—The Lord's Visit to Abraham and Sarah

1The Lord appeared to Abraham by the oaks of Mamre, as he sat at the
entrance of his tent in the heat of the day. 2He looked up and saw three
men standing near him. When he saw them, he ran from the tent entrance
to meet them, and bowed down to the ground. 3He said, "My lord, if I find
favor with you, do not pass by your servant. 4Let a little water be brought,
and wash your feet, and rest yourselves under the tree. 5Let me bring a
little bread, that you may refresh yourselves, and after that you may pass
on—since you have come to your servant." So they said, "Do as you have
said." 6And Abraham hastened into the tent to Sarah, and said, "Make
ready quickly three measures of choice flour, knead it, and make cakes."
7Abraham ran to the herd, and took a calf, tender and good, and gave it to
the servant, who hastened to prepare it. 8Then he took curds and milk and
the calf that he had prepared, and set it before them; and he stood by them
under the tree while they ate.

9They said to him, "Where is your wife Sarah?" And he said, "There, in
the tent." 10Then one said, "I will surely return to you in due season, and
your wife Sarah shall have a son." And Sarah was listening at the tent
entrance behind him. 11Now Abraham and Sarah were old, advanced in
age; it had ceased to be with Sarah after the manner of women. 12So Sarah
laughed to herself, saying, "After I have grown old, and my husband is
old, shall I have pleasure?" 13The Lord said to Abraham, "Why did Sarah
laugh, and say, 'Shall I indeed bear a child, now that I am old?' 14Is
anything too wonderful for the Lord? At the set time I will return to you,

in due season, and Sarah shall have a son." 15But Sarah denied, saying, "I
did not laugh"; for she was afraid. He said, "Oh yes, you did laugh."

Appendix B

Matthew 25:31–46—The Judgment

[31]When the Son of Man comes in his glory, and all the angels with him, then he will sit on the throne of his glory. [32]All the nations will be gathered before him, and he will separate people one from another as a shepherd separates the sheep from the goats, [33]and he will put the sheep at his right hand and the goats at the left. [34]Then the king will say to those at his right hand, "Come, you that are blessed by my Father, inherit the kingdom prepared for you from the foundation of the world; [35]for I was hungry and you gave me food, I was thirsty and you gave me something to drink, I was a stranger and you welcomed me, [36]I was naked and you gave me clothing, I was sick and you took care of me, I was in prison and you visited me." [37]Then the righteous will answer him, "Lord, when was it that we saw you hungry and gave you food, or thirsty and gave you something to drink? [38]And when was it that we saw you a stranger and welcomed you, or naked and gave you clothing? [39]And when was it that we saw you sick or in prison and visited you?" [40]And the king will answer them, "Truly I tell you, just as you did it to one of the least of these who are members of my family, you did it to me." [41]Then he will say to those at his left hand, "You that are accursed, depart from me into the eternal fire prepared for the devil and his angels; [42]for I was hungry and you gave me no food, I was thirsty and you gave me nothing to drink, [43]I was a stranger and you did not welcome me, naked and you did not give me clothing, sick and in prison and you did not visit me." [44]Then they also will answer, "Lord, when was it that we saw you hungry or thirsty or a stranger or naked or sick or in prison, and did not take care of you?" [45]Then he will answer them, "Truly I tell you, just as you did not do it to one of the least

of these, you did not do it to me." 46And these will go away into eternal punishment, but the righteous into eternal life.

Appendix C

Surah Al-Hijr 15:49–70

Tell My servants I am the All-forgiving, the All-compassionate, $_{49}$and that
My chastisement is the painful chastisement. $_{50}$And tell them of the guests of
Abraham, $_{51}$when they entered unto him, saying, “Peace!” He said, “Behold,
we are afraid of you.” $_{52}$They said, “Be not afraid; behold, we give thee good
tidings of a cunning boy.” $_{53}$He said, “What, do you give me good tidings,
though old age has smitten me? Of what do you $_{54}$give me good tidings?”
They said, “We give thee good tidings of truth. Be not of those that despair.”
$_{55}$He said, “And who despairs of the mercy of his Lord, excepting those that
are astray?” $_{56}$He said, “And what is your business, envoys?” $_{57}$They said,
“We have been sent unto a people of sinners, $_{58}$excepting the folk of Lot;
them we shall deliver $_{59}$all together, excepting his wife—we have decreed,
she shall surely be of those that tarry.” $_{60}$So, when the envoys came to the
folk of Lot, $_{61}$he said, “Surely you are a people unknown to me!” $_{62}$They said,
“Nay, but we have brought thee that concerning which they were doubting.
$_{63}$We have come to thee with the truth, and assuredly we speak truly. $_{64}$So set
forth, thou with thy family, in a watch of the night, and follow after the backs
of them, and let not any one of you turn round; and depart unto the place you
are commanded.” $_{65}$And We decreed for him that commandment, that the last
remnant of those should be cut off in the morning. $_{66}$And the people of the
city came rejoicing. $_{67}$He said, “These are my guests; put me not to shame,
$_{68}$and fear God, and do not degrade me.” $_{69}$They said, “Have we not forbidden
thee all beings?”$_{70}$

Appendix D

Surah Adh-Dhariyyat 51:22–37

And in heaven is your provision, and that you are promised. 22 So by the Lord
of heaven and earth, it is as surely true as that you have speech. 23 Hast thou
received the story of the honoured guests of Abraham? 24 When they entered
unto him, saying "Peace!" he said "Peace! You are a people unknown to
me." 25 Then he turned to his household and brought a fattened calf, 26 and he
laid it before them saying, "Will you not eat?" 27 Then he conceived a fear of
them. They said, "Be not afraid!" And they gave him good tidings of a
cunning boy. 28 Then came forward his wife, clamouring, and she smote her
face, and said, "An old woman, barren!" 29 They said, "So says thy Lord; He
is the All-wise, the All-knowing." 30 Said he, "And what is your business,
envoys?" 31 They said, "We have been sent to a people of sinners, 32 to loose
upon them stones of clay 33 marked with thy Lord for the prodigal. 34 So We
brought forth such believers as were in it, 35 but We found not therein except
one house of those that have surrendered themselves. 36 And therein We left a
sign to those who fear the painful chastisement." 37

Bibliography

Abd ‘Allah al-Khatib al-Tabrizi, Muhammad ibn. *Mishkat al-Masabih*, Vol. I, trans. James Robson (Islamabad, Pakistan: Orentalia Arts Ltd., 1999).

———. *Mishkat al-Masabih*, Vol. II, trans. James Robson (Islamabad, Pakistan: Orentalia Arts Ltd., 1999).

Akpinar, Snjezana. “Two Responses to ‘Interreligious Dialogue and Spiritual Hospitality’: Hospitality in Islam,” in *Religion East and West* 7 (2007): 23–27.

Alwy, Awliya and Susanne Schech. “Ethnic Inequalities in Education in Kenya.” *International Education Journal*, 5.2 (2004): 266–74.

Apostolic Exhortation on the Role of the Christian Family in the Modern World. *Familiaris Consortio* (Vatican: the Holy See, Rome, November 22, 1981).

Aquinas, Thomas. *Summa Theologica*, trans. Fathers of the English Dominican Province (Brewster, MA: Christian Classics, 1981).

Armstrong, Karen. *Muhammad: A Biography of the Prophet* (San Francisco, CA: Harper San Francisco, 1993).

Armstrong, Karen. *Islam: A Short History* (New York: Random House, Inc., 2000).

Asante, Molefi Kete and Abu S. Abarry. “Jomo Kenyatta, Religion and Ancestor Worship” in *African Intellectual Heritage: A Book of Sources*, eds. Molefi Kete Asante and Abu S. Abarry (Philadelphia: Temple University Press, 1996).

Ashforth, Adam. “An Epidemic of Witchcraft? The Implications of AIDS for the Post-Apartheid State.” *African Studies* 61.1 (2002): 121–43.

Augustine of Hippo. *The City of God*, trans. Marcus Dods DD (New York: The Modern Library).

Badri, Malik. “The AIDS Crisis: An Islamic Perspective,” in *Islam and AIDS: Between Scorn, Pity, and Justice*, eds. Farid Esack and Sarah Chiddy (Oxford, UK: Oneworld Publishing, 2009).

Becker, Felicitas. *Becoming Muslim in Mainland Tanzania, 1890–2000* (London, UK: Oxford University Press for the British Academy, 2008).

———. “Competing Explanations and Treatment Choices: Muslims, AIDS and ARVs in Tanzania,” in *AIDS and Religious Practice in Africa*, eds. Felicitas Becker and P. Wenzel Geissler (Leiden, Holland: E.J. Brill, 2009).

Browning, Melissa. “Theology and Morality on the Streets: An Examination of the Beliefs and Moral Formation of Street Children in Light of Christianity and African Traditional Religions,” in *Ethnography as Christian Theology and Ethics*, eds. Christian Scharen and Aana Marie Vigen (New York: Continuum International Publishing Group, 2011).

Bujo, Bénézet, SJ. “Community Ethics,” in *AIDS in Africa: Theological Reflections*, eds. Bénézet Bujo and Michael Czerny (Nairobi, Kenya: Paulines Publications Africa, 2007).

Burghardt, Marian. "Subjects of Counselling: Religion, HIV/AIDS and the Management of Everyday Life in South Africa," in *AIDS and Religious Practice in Africa*, eds. Felicitas Becker and P. Wenzel Geissler (Leiden, Holland: E.J. Brill, 2009).

Buysse, Caitlin Yoshiko. "The Qur'an, Poverty, and AIDS" in *Islam and AIDS: Between Scorn, Pity, and Justice*, eds. Farid Esack and Sarah Chiddy (Oxford, UK: Oneworld Publishing, 2009).

Cahill, Lisa Sowle. *Bioethics and the Common Good* (Milwaukee, WI: Marquette University Press, 2004).

———. *Theological Bioethics: Participation, Justice, and Change* (Washington, DC: Georgetown University Press, 2005).

Catholic Bishops of Africa and Madagascar. "KENYA, The Challenge of AIDS," in *Speak Out on HIV & AIDS* (Nairobi, Kenya: Paulines Publications Africa, 2006).

Catholic Church. *Catechism of the Catholic Church: Revised in Accordance with the Official Latin Text Promulgated by Pope John Paul II* (Vatican City, Libreria Editrice Vaticana, 1997).

Center for Disease Control (CDC). "Prevalence of Diagnosed and Undiagnosed HIV Infection—United States, 2008–2012," in *Morbidity and Mortality Weekly Report*, 63 (Atlanta: Center for Disease Control, 2015).

Central Intelligence Agency (CIA). "Africa—Kenya," in *The World Factbook 2003–14* (Washington, DC: Central Intelligence Agency, 2013).

Cornille, Catherine. *The Im-Possibility of Interreligious Dialogue* (New York: The Crossroads Publishing Company, 2008).

Czerny, Michael, SJ. "Working for Healing" in *AIDS in Africa: Theological Reflections*, eds. Bénézet Bujo and Michael Czerny (Nairobi, Kenya: Paulines Publications Africa, 2007).

Dilger, Hansjörg. "Sexuality, AIDS and the Lures of Modernity: Reflexivity and Morality among Young People in Rural Tanzania." *Medical Anthropology* 22.1. (2003): 23–52.

Dogmatic Constitution of the Church. *Lumen Gentium*. (Vatican: the Holy See, Rome, November 21, 1965).

Encyclical Letter on the Regulation of Birth. *Humanae Vitae*. (Vatican: the Holy See, Rome, July 25, 1968).

Esack, Farid. "Introduction," in *Islam and AIDS: Between Scorn, Pity, and Justice*, eds. Farid Esack and Sarah Chiddy (Oxford, UK: Oneworld Publishing, 2009).

———. "Practitioner Response," in *Religion and HIV and AIDS: Charting the Terrain*, ed. Beverly Haddad (Scottsville, South Africa: University of Kwazulu-Natal Press, 2011).

Farley, Margaret A. "How Shall We Love in a Postmodern World?" *The Annual of the Society of Christian Ethics* 14 (1994): 3–19.

———. *Just Love: A Framework for Christian Sexual Ethics* (London, UK: Continuum International Publishing Group, 2006).

———. *Compassionate Respect: A Feminist Approach to Medical Ethics and Other Questions* (Mahwah, NJ: Paulist Press, 2002).

Freeman-Grenville, G. S. P. "Al-Mas'udi: The Ivory Trade," in *The East African Coast: Selected Documents from the First to the Earlier Nineteenth Century*, comp. G. S. P. Freeman-Grenville (London UK: Oxford at the Clarendon Press, 1962).

———. "Vasco Da Gama's Discovery of East Africa for Portugal 1498," in *The East African Coast: Selected Documents from the First to the Earlier Nineteenth Century*, comp. G. S. P. Freeman-Grenville (London UK: Oxford at the Clarendon Press, 1962).

Fuller, Jon, SJ, and James Keenan, SJ. "Educating in a Time of HIV/AIDS: Learning from the Legacies of Human Rights, the Common Good, and the Works of Mercy," in *Opening Up: Speaking Out in the Church*, eds. Julian Filochowski and Peter Stanford (London, UK: Darton, Longman, & Todd, 2005).

Gaillardetz, Richard. *The Church in the Making: Lumen Gentium, Christus Dominus, Orientalium Ecclesiarum* (Mahwah, NJ: Paulist Press, 2006).

Geissler, P. Wenzel and Ruth Prince. *The Land is Dying: Contingency, Creativity, and Conflict in Western Kenya* (Oxford, UK: Berghahn Books, 2010).

Goldenberg, David A. *We Are all Brothers: The Suppression of Consciousness of Socio-Economic Differentiation in a Kenya Luo Lineage* (Ann Arbor, MI: University Microfilms, Int'l, 1982).

Gray, Peter B. "HIV and Islam: Is HIV Prevalence Lower among Muslims?" *Social Science and Medicine* 58.9 (2004): 1751–56.

Herbermann, Charles G., Edward A. Pace, Condé B. Pallen, Thomas J. Shahan, and John J. Wynne, SJ, eds. *The Catholic Encyclopedia: An International Work of Reference on the Constitution, Doctrine, Discipline, and History of the Catholic Church*, Vol. 1 (New York: The Encyclopedia Press, Inc., 1913).

Hinga, Teresia Mbari. "Africa's Transformative Responses to the Gendered Global HIV and AIDS Syndemic." *HIV and AIDS in Africa: Christian Reflection, Public Health, Social Transformation*, ed. Jacquineau Azetsop, SJ (Maryknoll, NY: Orbis Books, 2016).

———. "AIDS, Religion and Women in Africa: Theo-Ethical Challenges and Imperatives," in *Women, Religion and HIV and AIDS in Africa: Responding to Ethical and Theological Challenges*, ed. Teresia Mbari Hinga et al. (Pietermaritzburg, South Africa: Cluster Publications, 2008).

Hirtenstein, Stephen and Martin Notcutt. *Divine Sayings: 101 Hadith Qudsi* (Oxford, UK: Anqa Publishing, 2008)

Holy Bible. *The New Oxford Annotated Bible: New Revised Standard Version with the Apocrypha*, ed. Michael D. Coogan (New York: Oxford University Press, 2001).

Holy Qur'ān. *The Koran Interpreted: A Translation*, trans. A. J. Arberry (New York: Touchstone, 1996).

Joint United Nations Programme on HIV/AIDS (UNAIDS). *Global Report: UNAIDS Report on the Global AIDS Epidemic 2013* (Geneva, Switzerland: UNAIDS Secretariat, 2013).

———. *UNAIDS Data 2017* (Geneva, Switzerland: UNAIDS Secretariat, 2017).

Keenan, James F., SJ. *The Works of Mercy: The Heart of Catholicism* (Lanham, MD: Rowman and Littlefield Publishers, 2007).

Keenan, James F., SJ, and Jon D. Fuller, SJ. "Condoms, Catholics and HIV/AIDS Prevention." *The Furrow* 52.9 (2001): 459–67.

Kelly, Kevin. "Conclusion: A Moral Theologian Faces the New Millennium in a Time of AIDS" in *Catholic Ethicists on HIV/AIDS Prevention*, eds. James F. Keenan, Jon Fuller, SJ, Lisa Cahill, and Kevin Kelly (New York: Continuum Books, 2000).

Kelly, Michael J., SJ. *HIV and AIDS: A Social Justice Perspective* (Nairobi, Kenya: Paulines Publications Africa, 2010).

Kenyan Episcopal Conference (KEC). "The Church Presents Her Strategy," in *This We Teach and Do: Catholic Church and AIDS in Kenya*, Vol. 1—*Policy* (Nairobi, Kenya: Paulines Publications Africa, 2006).

———. "The Church Speaks and Teaches," in *This We Teach and Do: Catholic Church and AIDS in Kenya*, Vol. 1—*Policy* (Nairobi, Kenya: Paulines Publications Africa, 2006).

———. "Foreword," in *This We Teach and Do: Catholic Church and AIDS in Kenya*, Vol. 1—*Policy* (Nairobi, Kenya: Paulines Publications Africa, 2006).

Khan, Jamal Nasir, Sukhmeet Singh Panesar, Abdul Rashid Gatrad, and Aziz Sheikh. "The Cross, the Crescent, and the Contagion: Ecological Study of the Association between Religious Affiliation to Christianity and Islam, and Adult Prevalence of HIV/AIDS in Africa." *Journal of the Islamic Medical Association of South Africa* 12.1 (2005): 17–18.

Knox, Peter, SJ. *AIDS, Ancestors, and Salvation* (Nairobi, Kenya: Paulines Publications Africa, 2005).

Kollman, Paul V. *The Evangelization of Slaves and Catholic Origins in Eastern Africa* (Maryknoll, NY: Orbis Books, 2005).

Kragh, Simon U. "The Anthropology of Nepotism: Social Distance and Reciprocity in Organizations in Developing Countries." *International Journal of Cross Cultural Management* 12.2 (2012): 247–65.

Laws of Kenya. *Penal Code of 1930* (Nairobi, Kenya: Government Printers, rev. ed. 2012).

Leebaw, Bronwyn. "Legitimation or Judgment? South Africa's Restorative Approach to Transitional Justice. *Polity* 36.1 (October 2003): 23–51.

Library of Congress. *Laws on Homosexuality in African Nations* (Washington, DC: The Law Library of Congress, 2014).

Magesa, Laurenti. "Contextualizing HIV and AIDS in the African Reality," in *HIV and AIDS in Africa: Christian Reflection, Public Health, Social Transformation*, ed. Jacquineau Azetsop, SJ (Maryknoll, NY: Orbis Books, 2016).

Maritain, Jacques. *The Person and the Common Good* (South Bend, IN: University of Notre Dame Press, 1947).

McDermott, J. Michael, SJ. "Is AIDS God's Punishment?" *Homiletic & Pastoral Review*, 32 (1991), 32–58.

McIntosh, Janet. *The Edge of Islam: Power, Personhood, and Ethnoreligious Boundaries on the Kenyan Coast* (Durham, NC: Duke University Press, 2009).

Messer, Donald E. *Breaking the Conspiracy of Silence: Christian Churches and the Global AIDS* Crisis (Minneapolis: Fortress Press, 2004).

Mkenda, Festo, SJ. "Of Things Old and New: The African Sociohistorical Context of an HIV-and-AIDS Theology," in *HIV and AIDS in Africa: Christian Reflection, Public Health, Social Transformation*, ed. Jacquineau Azetsop, SJ (Maryknoll, NY: Orbis Books, 2016).

Morris, James W. *Openings: From the Qur'an to the Islamic Humanities* (Personal Manuscript, 2010).

Murata, Sachiko and William Chittick. *The Vision of Islam* (St. Paul, MN: Paragon House, 1994).

National AIDS Control Council (NACC). *Kenya AIDS Response Progress Report, 2014: Progress Towards Zero* (Nairobi, Kenya: National AIDS Control Council of Kenya, 2014).

National Council for Law Reporting. *The Constitution of Kenya* (Nairobi, Kenya: Kenyan National Legislative Bodies, August 27, 2010).

Niehaus, Isak. "Leprosy of a Deadlier Kind: Christian Conceptions of AIDS in the South African Lowveld, in *AIDS and Religious Practice in Africa*, eds. Felicitas Becker and P. Wenzel Geissler (Leiden, Holland: E.J. Brill, 2009).

Nurse, Derek and Thomas Spear. *The Swahili: Reconstructing the History and Language of an African Society, 800–1500* (Philadelphia: University of Pennsylvania Press, 1985).

Nzioka, Charles, Allan Korongo, and Roseanne Njiru. *HIV and AIDS in Kenyan Teacher Colleges: Mitigating the Impact* (Paris, France: International Institute for Educational Planning, 2007).

Oketch, Moses and Caine Rolleston. "Policies on Free Primary Secondary Education in East Africa: Retrospect and Prospect," *Journal of Research in Education* 31 (2007): 131–58.

Orobator, Agbonkhianmeghe E., SJ. *From Crisis to Kairos*: *The Mission of the Church in the Time of HIV/AIDS, Refugees, and Poverty* (Nairobi, Kenya: Paulines Publications Africa, 2005).

———. "When AIDS Comes to Church" in *AIDS in Africa: Theological Reflections*, eds. Bénézet Bujo and Michael Czerny (Nairobi, Kenya: Paulines Publications Africa, 2007).

Otieno, Adam. "Drug Abuse in Kisumu Town, Western Kenya." *African Journal of Food, Agriculture, Nutrition, and Development* 9:3 (2009), 1–10.

Paterson, Gillian. *Stigma in the Context of Development* (London, UK: Progressio, 2009).

Pope Benedict XVI. "Healing and Forming the Whole Person" in *AIDS in Africa: Theological Reflections*, eds. Bénézet Bujo and Michael Czerny (Nairobi, Kenya: Paulines Publications Africa, 2007).

Pope John Paul II. "Christ, Hope for Africa—Message for the 13th World Day of the Sick," in Catholic Bishops of Africa and Madagascar, *Speak out on HIV & AIDS* (Nairobi, Kenya: Paulines Publications Africa, 2006).

Pouwels, Randall L. *Horn and Crescent: Cultural Exchange and Traditional Islam on the East African Coast, 800–1900* (New York: Cambridge University Press, 1987).

Prince, Ruth. "Christian Salvation and Luo Tradition: Arguments of Faith in a Time of Death in Western Kenya," in *AIDS and Religious Practice in Africa*, eds. Felicitas Becker and P. Wenzel Geissler (Leiden, Holland: E.J. Brill, 2009).

Sachedina, Abdulaziz. *Islamic Biomedical Ethics: Principles and Applications* (New York: Oxford University Press, 2009).

Sadgrove, Jo. " 'Keeping Up Appearances': Sex and Religion Amongst University Students in Uganda" in *AIDS and Religious Practice in Africa*, eds. Felicitas Becker and P. Wenzel Geissler (Leiden, Holland: E.J. Brill, 2009).

Shah-Kazemi, Reza. *My Mercy Encompasses All Things: The Koran's Teaching on Compassion, Peace, and Love* (Berkeley, CA: Counterpoint, 2007).

Snidle, Heather and David Yeoman. *Christ in AIDS: An Educational, Pastoral and Spiritual Approach to HIV/AIDS* (Cardiff, UK: Cardiff Academic Press, 1997).

Stark, Rodney. *The Rise of Christianity: How the Obscure, Marginal Jesus Movement Became the Dominant Religious Force in the Western World in a Few Centuries* (San Francisco, CA: Harper San Francisco, 1997).

Strathdee, Steffanie A., Timothy B. Hallett, Natalia Bobrova, Tim Rhodes, Robert Booth, Reychad Abdool, Catherine A. Hankins. "HIV and Risk Environment for Injecting Drug Users: The Past, Present, and Future." *The Lancet* 376 (2010): 268–84.

Svensson, Johannes. " 'Muslims Have Instructions': HIV/AIDS, Modernity and Islamic Religious Education in Kisumu, Kenya," in *AIDS and Religious Practice in Africa*, eds. Felicitas Becker and P. Wenzel Geissler (Leiden, Holland: E.J. Brill, 2009).

Thompson, Vincent Bakpetu. *Conflict in the Horn of Africa: The Kenya-Somali Border Problem 1941–2014* (Lanham, MD: UPA Publications, 2015).

Tribble, Jeffrey L. "Ethnographic Research on African Pastoral Leadership and Congregations," in *Ethnography as Christian Theology and Ethics*, eds. Christian Scharen and Aana Marie Vigen (New York: Continuum International Publishing Group, 2011).

Turner, Victor. *The Ritual Process: Structure and Anti-Structure* (Piscataway, NJ: Aldine Transaction, Reprint Edition, 1995).

U.S. President's Emergency Plan for AIDS Relief (PEPFAR). *Kenya—Country Operational Plan—FY 2014* (Washington, DC: Office of the U.S. Global AIDS Coordinator and Health Diplomacy).

van Dijk, Rijk. "Gloves in the Time of AIDS: Pentecostalism, Hair, and Social Distancing in Botswana" in *AIDS and Religious Practice in Africa*, eds. Felicitas Becker and P. Wenzel Geissler (Leiden, Holland: E.J. Brill, 2009).

Watkins, Claire. "Organizing the People of God: Social-Science Theories of Organization in Ecclesiology," *Theological Studies* 52 (1991).

Whitehouse, David. "East Africa and the Maritime Trade of the Indian Ocean, AD 800–1500," in *Islam in East Africa; New Sources*, ed. Biancamaria Amoretti (Rome, Italy: International Colloquium, 2001).

Worell, Judith, ed. *Encyclopedia of Women and Gender: Sex Similarities and Differences and the Impact of Society on Gender*, Vol. 2 (Waltham, MA: Academic Press Publishing Company, 2001).

Ziraba, Abdhalah Kasiira, Catherine Kyobutungi, and Eliya Msiyaphazi Zulu. "Fatal Injuries in the Slums of Nairobi and their Risk Factors: Results from a Matched Case-Control Study." *Journal of Urban Health: Bulletin of the New York Academy of Medicine* 88, suppl. 2 (2011): 256–65.

Index

About the Author

Timothy James Carey received his doctorate in comparative theology at Boston College in Chestnut Hill, Massachusetts, where he studied Muslim-Christian relations in sub-Saharan Africa. His current research examines the respective Sunni Muslim and African Catholic responses to the HIV/AIDS pandemic in Nairobi, Kenya, as a case study for practical interreligious dialogue. His article on the influence of *Gaudium et Spes* and *Lumen Gentium* on the African Synods was published recently in the *Dharmaram Journal of Theology*. He is currently working on a project for the journal, *Theology and Sexuality,* on Muslim and Catholic efforts in the area of HIV/AIDS prevention and education in Nairobi, Kenya.

Lightning Source UK Ltd.
Milton Keynes UK
UKHW04n1112240918
329305UK00007B/39/P

9 781498 578288